Heal Your Gut, Heal Your Life

A Comprehensive Guide to Gut Recovery

COPYRIGHT

TABLE OF CONTENTS

INTRODUCTION

Deep within your body, an incredible world exists, one filled with intrigue and wonder. It's not a destination you can travel to, but rather a realm that resides within you, within your gut. Your gut, often underappreciated and understated, is a thriving ecosystem of microorganisms and processes that profoundly influence your health, happiness, and vitality.

Your gut is no ordinary organ—it's a powerhouse, a microcosm that influences nearly every aspect of your life. And yet, it often remains in the shadows, uncelebrated for the superhero that it is. The truth is, your gut is the epicenter of your health, a linchpin that connects body and mind in ways you might not have realized.

The importance of gut health cannot be overstated. It's not just about digestion; it's about your immune system, your mental well-being, and your overall quality of life. Every morsel you eat, every emotion you feel, and every day you wake up—your gut is there, orchestrating a silent symphony that shapes your world.

This guide is your portal into the captivating universe of gut health and a testament to the astonishing ways it shapes your life. You may have heard the phrase "trust your gut," but the truth is, your gut is the very core of trust when it comes to your overall well-being.

In a world dominated by quick fixes and external remedies, it's easy to forget that true health begins from within, within the remarkable intricacies of your gastrointestinal system. Your gut is more than a mere food processor; it is a dynamic organ that connects your body and mind, affecting everything from digestion to immunity, mood, metabolism, and even your susceptibility to chronic diseases.

The central character in this story is the gut microbiome, an army of trillions of microorganisms residing in your intestines. These tiny inhabitants are more than just passengers; they are active participants in your daily life, orchestrating a symphony that can determine your energy levels, emotional state, and long-term well-being.

The significance of gut health is not confined to the realm of science; it's a personal journey that each of us must undertake. It's about taking charge of your health, understanding the nuances of your body, and embracing the empowerment that comes with it. Your gut has the potential to be your silent partner, working relentlessly in the background to support and nurture you.

This guide is your path to unveiling the gut's hidden power, understanding its pivotal role in your life, and providing you with the tools and knowledge to nurture it. We will explore the science behind gut health and delve into the practical steps you can take to optimize your gut and, in turn, enhance your life.

From understanding the gut's role in digestive health to unlocking its secrets in the realms of mental clarity, immunity, and long-term well-being, this guide is your comprehensive resource. It aims to educate, inspire, and equip you with actionable strategies, whether you're seeking relief from digestive discomfort, fortifying your immune system, or simply yearning for more vitality and vigor.

CHAPTER ONE

Gut health refers to the well-being and optimal functioning of the gastrointestinal system, which includes the stomach, small intestine, large intestine, and associated organs. It is a crucial aspect of overall health and has a profound impact on various bodily functions. Here's an overview of gut health, its importance, and its role in overall well-being:

1. Anatomy and Functions of the Gastrointestinal System:

The gastrointestinal (GI) system is a complex and highly organized network of organs responsible for digesting food, absorbing nutrients, and eliminating waste.

Key components of the GI system include the mouth, esophagus, stomach, small intestine, large intestine, liver, gallbladder, and pancreas.

Functions of the GI system include breaking down food, extracting nutrients, protecting against harmful microorganisms, and eliminating waste.

2. The Gut Microbiome:

The gut is home to trillions of microorganisms, including bacteria, viruses, and fungi. These microorganisms make up the gut microbiome, a dynamic ecosystem that plays a pivotal role in digestion, immunity, and overall health.

A balanced and diverse gut microbiome is essential for optimal functioning. It helps digest certain foods, synthesizes vitamins, and protects against harmful pathogens.

3. Importance of Gut Health:

Gut health is linked to numerous aspects of well-being, including digestion, nutrient absorption, immunity, and mental health.

A healthy gut microbiome can contribute to reduced inflammation, better metabolic health, and a reduced risk of chronic diseases.

4. Common Digestive Problems:

Gastrointestinal issues are prevalent and can affect people of all ages. Some common digestive problems include irritable bowel syndrome (IBS), acid reflux, constipation, diarrhea, and inflammatory bowel diseases (IBD) such as Crohn's disease and ulcerative colitis.

5. Diet and Gut Health:

Diet plays a crucial role in gut health. Consuming a diet rich in fiber, whole foods, and probiotics can support a diverse and balanced gut microbiome.

Processed foods, excessive sugar, and artificial additives can disrupt the gut microbiome and lead to digestive problems.

6. Gut-Friendly Foods:

Gut-friendly foods include fiber-rich fruits and vegetables, whole grains, legumes, lean proteins, yogurt, kefir, and fermented foods. These foods promote gut health and support beneficial gut bacteria.

7. Supplements and Probiotics:

Supplements such as probiotics, prebiotics, and digestive enzymes can be used to support gut health, but they should be taken thoughtfully and with guidance from healthcare professionals.

8. Lifestyle Factors:

Lifestyle factors like stress management, regular exercise, sufficient sleep, and reduced alcohol and tobacco use play a significant role in maintaining gut health.

9. Reintroducing Foods and Tracking Progress:

After an elimination phase, reintroducing certain foods gradually and tracking your body's responses can help identify specific dietary triggers.

10. Long-Term Gut Health:

Maintaining long-term gut health requires consistency in healthy dietary and lifestyle habits. Regular check-ups and periodic assessments of gut health can be beneficial.

11. Seek Professional Guidance:

If you have specific gut health concerns, chronic digestive conditions, or food allergies, consider seeking guidance from healthcare professionals or registered dietitians to develop a personalized plan for optimal gut health.

In summary, gut health is a holistic concept that encompasses the digestive system, the gut microbiome, and the interplay between diet, lifestyle, and overall well-being. It's a dynamic aspect of health that can be nurtured and maintained to support optimal physical and mental health throughout one's life.

THE ANATOMY AND FUNCTIONS OF THE GASTROINTESTINAL SYSTEM.

The gastrointestinal system, often referred to as the digestive system, is a complex and vital organ system responsible for processing the food we eat, extracting nutrients, and eliminating waste products. It consists of various organs and tissues working in coordination to facilitate the digestion and absorption of nutrients. Here's an overview of the anatomy and functions of the gastrointestinal system:

Anatomy of the Gastrointestinal System:

• Mouth: Digestion begins in the mouth, where food is broken down mechanically by chewing and chemically through the action of salivary enzymes.

• Esophagus: The esophagus is a muscular tube that transports chewed food from the mouth to the stomach through a series of coordinated contractions called peristalsis.

• Stomach: The stomach serves as a storage and mixing chamber. It secretes gastric juices, including hydrochloric acid and digestive enzymes, which help break down food into a semi-liquid mixture called chyme.

• Small Intestine: The small intestine is where most digestion and nutrient absorption occur. It comprises three parts: the duodenum, jejunum, and ileum. Here, digestive enzymes from the pancreas and bile from the liver further break down food, and the resulting nutrients are absorbed through the intestinal lining into the bloodstream.

• Liver: The liver is a large organ that produces bile, a greenish fluid that helps emulsify fats, making them easier to digest. The liver also plays a crucial role in metabolizing nutrients and detoxifying the body.

• Gallbladder: The gallbladder stores and concentrates bile produced by the liver. When needed, it releases bile into the small intestine to aid in fat digestion.

• Pancreas: The pancreas secretes digestive enzymes (such as amylase, lipase, and proteases) into the small intestine to break down carbohydrates, fats, and proteins. It also releases insulin and glucagon to regulate blood sugar levels.

• Large Intestine (Colon): The large intestine is primarily responsible for water and electrolyte absorption, leading to the formation of feces. It houses a diverse community of bacteria that further break down undigested materials and synthesize certain vitamins.

• Rectum: The rectum serves as a temporary storage site for feces before elimination.

• Anus: The anus is the final part of the gastrointestinal system and is equipped with sphincters that control the expulsion of feces from the body.

Functions of the Gastrointestinal System:

• Ingestion: The process of taking food and liquids into the mouth.

• Digestion: The mechanical and chemical breakdown of food into smaller, absorbable components. Mechanical digestion includes chewing and stomach churning, while chemical digestion involves enzymes and acids breaking down macronutrients (carbohydrates, proteins, and fats).

• Absorption: The uptake of nutrients (such as amino acids, sugars, fatty acids, and vitamins) into the bloodstream from the small intestine's walls.

• Motility: The movement of food and waste products through the digestive tract, facilitated by muscular contractions (peristalsis).

• Secretion: The release of digestive juices, including stomach acid, bile, and pancreatic enzymes, to aid in digestion.

• Storage and Mixing: The stomach and large intestine function as storage and mixing chambers, ensuring a controlled release of digested food into the small intestine.

• Elimination: The expulsion of indigestible food residues and waste products (feces) through the rectum and anus.

The gastrointestinal system is a highly coordinated and essential system that sustains life by providing the body with the nutrients it needs while safely eliminating waste products.

Proper function of this system is crucial for overall health and well-being.

THE GUT MICROBIOME

The gut microbiome, also known as the gut microbiota, refers to the diverse community of microorganisms that inhabit the gastrointestinal tract, particularly the large intestine (colon). These microorganisms include bacteria, viruses, fungi, and other single-celled organisms. The gut microbiome plays a crucial role in human health and has garnered significant attention in recent years due to its influence on various aspects of well-being. Here are some key characteristics and functions of the gut microbiome:

1. Diversity: The gut microbiome is highly diverse, with trillions of microorganisms belonging to thousands of different species. This diversity is essential for maintaining a balanced and healthy microbiome.

2. Symbiotic Relationship: Humans and their gut microbiota have a mutualistic relationship, meaning both parties benefit. The microbiota helps with various aspects of digestion and

provides other health-related functions in exchange for the nutrients and environment the human host provides.

3. Digestive Aid: The gut microbiome aids in the digestion of certain foods and the absorption of nutrients. It breaks down complex carbohydrates, ferments fibers, and helps metabolize fats and proteins that the human body alone cannot efficiently process.

4. Immune System Support: A significant portion of the immune system is influenced by the gut microbiome. It helps protect against harmful pathogens, regulates the immune response, and maintains a balance between inflammation and tolerance.

5. Synthesis of Vitamins and Short-Chain Fatty Acids: Some gut bacteria synthesize essential vitamins (e.g., vitamin K and certain B vitamins) and produce short-chain fatty acids (SCFAs) that serve as an energy source for the colon and have various health benefits.

6. Gut-Brain Axis: Emerging research suggests that the gut microbiome can influence brain function and mental health through the gut-brain axis. Changes in the microbiome

composition have been linked to conditions like depression and anxiety.

7. Metabolism and Weight Regulation: The gut microbiome may play a role in regulating metabolism and body weight. Imbalances in the microbiome have been associated with obesity and metabolic disorders.

8. Protection Against Pathogens: The gut microbiome can inhibit the growth of harmful pathogens by competing for nutrients and producing antimicrobial compounds.

9. Influences on Systemic Health: Research has linked the gut microbiome to a range of systemic health conditions, including autoimmune diseases, allergies, and even cardiovascular health.

10. Individual Variation: Each person's gut microbiome is unique, influenced by factors like genetics, diet, environment, and early-life exposures, such as birth method (vaginal or Cesarean) and breastfeeding.

The gut microbiome is a dynamic and adaptable ecosystem that can change over time in response to various factors, including diet, antibiotics, and lifestyle choices. Maintaining a balanced and diverse gut microbiome is associated with better health outcomes, while imbalances or disruptions in the microbiome, often referred to as dysbiosis, can lead to various health issues. Researchers continue to explore the role of the gut microbiome in health and disease, offering new insights into personalized medicine and potential interventions for improving health.

THE ROLE OF GUT MICROBIOME IN OVERALL HEALTH

The gut microbiome plays a pivotal role in overall health, influencing various aspects of physical and even mental well-being. Its impact on human health is a dynamic and evolving field of research. Here are some of the key roles the gut microbiome plays in maintaining and promoting overall health:

1. Digestion and Nutrient Absorption: The gut microbiome is essential for breaking down complex carbohydrates, fibers, and other substances in food that the human body cannot digest on its own. It helps convert these compounds into absorbable nutrients, such as short-chain fatty acids (SCFAs), which provide an energy source for the colon and play a role in metabolic health.

2. Immune System Regulation: A significant portion of the immune system is located in the gut-associated lymphoid tissue (GALT), and the gut microbiome helps regulate immune function. It assists in distinguishing between beneficial microorganisms and harmful pathogens, promoting tolerance to harmless antigens and initiating immune responses when needed.

3. Protection Against Pathogens: The gut microbiome competes with and inhibits the growth of harmful pathogens by consuming available nutrients and producing antimicrobial compounds. This defense mechanism helps maintain gut health and prevents infections.

4. Synthesis of Essential Nutrients: Some gut bacteria synthesize essential vitamins (e.g., vitamin K and certain B vitamins) that the human body cannot produce on its own. This ensures a steady supply of these vital nutrients for overall health.

5. Metabolism and Weight Regulation: Research suggests that the gut microbiome can influence metabolism and body weight. Imbalances in the microbiome composition have been linked to obesity and metabolic disorders, while a balanced

microbiome may help regulate appetite and promote a healthy weight.

6. Gut-Brain Axis: The gut microbiome communicates with the brain through the gut-brain axis, potentially influencing mood, behavior, and cognitive function. Imbalances in the gut microbiome have been associated with mental health conditions such as depression, anxiety, and even neurodegenerative diseases.

7. Systemic Health Implications: Dysbiosis, or an imbalance in the gut microbiome, has been linked to various health conditions beyond the gut, including autoimmune diseases, allergies, cardiovascular health, and more. Research continues to uncover the connections between the gut microbiome and systemic health.

8. Detoxification: Some gut bacteria aid in the detoxification of harmful substances, promoting the body's ability to eliminate toxins.

9. Influence of Medications: The gut microbiome can affect the metabolism and effectiveness of certain medications, including

drugs used for cardiovascular health and mental health conditions.

10. Influence of Diet and Lifestyle: Dietary choices, lifestyle factors (e.g., physical activity, stress management), and medications can all impact the composition and diversity of the gut microbiome. Making healthy choices can promote a more diverse and balanced gut microbiome, which is associated with better health outcomes.

11. Personalized Medicine: Understanding an individual's gut microbiome can be a part of personalized medicine. It can help tailor dietary recommendations, treatments, and interventions to optimize health based on a person's unique microbiome profile.

The gut microbiome is a complex and dynamic ecosystem that responds to a variety of factors, including diet, genetics, environment, and early-life exposures. Maintaining a diverse and balanced gut microbiome is associated with better health outcomes, while disruptions can lead to various health issues. Ongoing research is shedding light on the immense potential for interventions aimed at optimizing gut health to improve overall well-being.

Digestive problems, also known as gastrointestinal disorders, can range from mild and temporary to severe and chronic. These conditions can affect various parts of the gastrointestinal tract and may result from a variety of factors, including diet, lifestyle, genetics, and infections. Here are some common digestive problems, along with explanations for each:

1. Gastroesophageal Reflux Disease (GERD): GERD is a chronic condition in which stomach acid flows back into the esophagus, causing symptoms such as heartburn, regurgitation, and chest pain. Over time, it can lead to inflammation and damage to the esophagus lining.

2. Irritable Bowel Syndrome (IBS): IBS is a functional gastrointestinal disorder characterized by abdominal pain, bloating, and changes in bowel habits, such as diarrhea, constipation, or alternating between the two. It does not cause structural damage to the digestive tract but can significantly impact quality of life.

3. Inflammatory Bowel Disease (IBD): IBD encompasses two main conditions: Crohn's disease and ulcerative colitis. These are chronic autoimmune disorders that cause inflammation and damage to the gastrointestinal tract. Symptoms include diarrhea, abdominal pain, weight loss, and fatigue.

4. Celiac Disease: Celiac disease is an autoimmune disorder triggered by the consumption of gluten, a protein found in wheat, barley, and rye. It damages the lining of the small intestine, leading to malabsorption of nutrients. Symptoms may include diarrhea, abdominal pain, fatigue, and weight loss.

5. Gallstones: Gallstones are hard, pebble-like deposits that form in the gallbladder. They can block the flow of bile, causing pain in the upper abdomen, known as biliary colic. If they obstruct the bile duct, it can lead to inflammation (cholecystitis) and complications.

6. Constipation: Constipation is a common digestive issue characterized by infrequent and difficult bowel movements. It can result from various factors, including a low-fiber diet, dehydration, and certain medications.

7. Diarrhea: Diarrhea involves frequent, loose, or watery bowel movements. It can be caused by infections, food intolerances, medications, or underlying medical conditions.

8. Peptic Ulcers: Peptic ulcers are open sores that develop on the inner lining of the stomach (gastric ulcers) or the upper part of the small intestine (duodenal ulcers). They can cause abdominal pain, bloating, and bleeding in severe cases.

9. Diverticulitis: Diverticulitis is the inflammation or infection of small pouches (diverticula) that can form in the colon. Symptoms include abdominal pain, fever, and changes in bowel habits.

10. Gastroenteritis: Gastroenteritis is often referred to as the stomach flu. It is an infection or inflammation of the stomach and intestines, causing symptoms such as diarrhea, vomiting, abdominal cramps, and nausea.

11. Lactose Intolerance: Lactose intolerance is the inability to digest lactose, a sugar found in milk and dairy products. Symptoms include bloating, diarrhea, and abdominal pain after consuming lactose-containing foods.

12. Pancreatitis: Pancreatitis is the inflammation of the pancreas, which can result from gallstones, alcohol consumption, or other factors. It causes severe abdominal pain, nausea, and vomiting.

13. Gastrointestinal Cancers: Conditions such as stomach cancer, colorectal cancer, and pancreatic cancer can affect the gastrointestinal tract. Symptoms vary but may include unexplained weight loss, abdominal pain, and changes in bowel habits.

It's important to note that if you experience persistent or severe digestive symptoms, it's advisable to consult a healthcare professional for proper diagnosis and treatment. Many digestive problems can be managed or even prevented with dietary and lifestyle changes, medications, and, in some cases, surgical interventions.

SYMPTOMS OF THE COMMON DIGESTIVE PROBLEMS LISTED ABOVE

Here are some common symptoms associated with the digestive problems listed above:

• Heartburn (burning sensation in the chest)

• Regurgitation (acid or food flowing back into the mouth)

• Chest pain

• Difficulty swallowing (dysphagia)

Irritable Bowel Syndrome (IBS):

• Abdominal pain or discomfort

• Bloating and gas

• Altered bowel habits (diarrhea, constipation, or alternating between the two)

• Mucus in the stool

• Urgency to have a bowel movement

Inflammatory Bowel Disease (IBD):

• Diarrhea

• Abdominal pain and cramps

- Weight loss

- Fatigue

- Bloody stools (ulcerative colitis)

- Skip lesions, fissures, and strictures (Crohn's disease)

Celiac Disease:

- Diarrhea

- Abdominal pain and bloating

- Fatigue

- Skin rashes

- Unexplained weight loss

Gallstones:

- Biliary colic (intense pain in the upper right abdomen or upper back)

- Nausea and vomiting

- Jaundice (yellowing of the skin and eyes) in severe cases

Constipation:

• Infrequent bowel movements (typically fewer than three per week)

• Hard, dry stools

• Straining during bowel movements

• A feeling of incomplete evacuation

Diarrhea:

• Frequent, loose, or watery bowel movements

• Urgency to have a bowel movement

• Abdominal cramps

• Bloating and gas

Peptic Ulcers:

• Burning or gnawing abdominal pain, often between meals and at night

• Bloating and burping

• Nausea

• Dark, tarry stools (if there is bleeding)

• Lower left abdominal pain, often severe

• Fever

• Changes in bowel habits

• Bloating and cramps

• Diarrhea

• Vomiting

• Abdominal cramps

• Nausea

• Bloating

• Diarrhea

• Abdominal cramps

• Gas

Pancreatitis:

• Severe, piercing abdominal pain

• Nausea and vomiting

• Fever

• Rapid pulse

Gastrointestinal Cancers: Symptoms can vary depending on the specific type and stage of cancer but may include unexplained weight loss, abdominal pain, changes in bowel habits, blood in the stool, and fatigue.

Please note that these symptoms are general descriptions, and individual experiences can vary. If you experience persistent or severe symptoms, or if you have concerns about your digestive health, it's important to seek medical advice for a proper diagnosis and appropriate treatment.

Here are some potential causes for the common digestive problems listed above:

Gastroesophageal Reflux Disease (GERD):

• Weak Lower Esophageal Sphincter (LES): The LES, which separates the esophagus from the stomach, may not close properly, allowing stomach acid to flow back into the esophagus.

• Hiatal Hernia: When part of the stomach protrudes through the diaphragm, it can weaken the LES.

Irritable Bowel Syndrome (IBS): The exact cause of IBS is not fully understood, but it may involve a combination of factors, including altered gut motility, heightened sensitivity of the intestines, infections, and disturbances in the gut-brain axis.

Inflammatory Bowel Disease (IBD):

• Autoimmune Response: IBD is believed to result from an abnormal immune response, where the body's immune system attacks the digestive tract.

• Genetic Factors: There is a genetic predisposition to IBD.

• Environmental Factors: Infections or environmental triggers can play a role.

Celiac Disease:

Immune Reaction to Gluten: Celiac disease is triggered by an autoimmune response to the ingestion of gluten-containing foods (wheat, barley, rye) in genetically predisposed individuals.

Gallstones:

• Cholesterol or Pigment Stones: Gallstones can form when there's an imbalance in the substances that make up bile, leading to the formation of cholesterol or pigment stones.

• Gallbladder Dysfunction: Gallbladder motility issues can contribute to stone formation.

Constipation:

• Low Fiber Diet: Diets low in fiber can lead to infrequent bowel movements and difficulty passing stools.

• Dehydration: Insufficient fluid intake can lead to hard, dry stools and constipation.

• Lifestyle Factors: Lack of physical activity and delaying the urge to have a bowel movement can contribute to constipation.

Diarrhea:

• Infections: Bacterial, viral, or parasitic infections can lead to acute diarrhea.

• Food Intolerances: Intolerance to certain foods, such as lactose or gluten, can cause chronic diarrhea.

• Irritable Bowel Syndrome: Diarrhea-predominant IBS can result in recurrent bouts of diarrhea.

Peptic Ulcers:

• Helicobacter pylori Infection: Infection with H. pylori bacteria is a common cause of peptic ulcers.

• Nonsteroidal Anti-Inflammatory Drugs (NSAIDs): The chronic use of NSAIDs like aspirin or ibuprofen can contribute to ulcer formation.

Diverticulitis:

• Formation of Diverticula: Small pouches (diverticula) can form in the colon over time, particularly when there is a low-fiber diet.

• Infection or Inflammation: When these pouches become infected or inflamed, diverticulitis can occur.

Gastroenteritis:

• Infections: Gastroenteritis is often caused by viral, bacterial, or parasitic infections, such as norovirus or E. coli.

Lactose Intolerance:

• Lactase Deficiency: Lactose intolerance occurs when the body does not produce enough of the enzyme lactase, which is needed to digest lactose.

Pancreatitis:

• Gallstones: Pancreatitis can result from gallstones blocking the pancreatic duct.

• Alcohol Abuse: Chronic alcohol consumption is a common cause of pancreatitis.

• High Triglyceride Levels: Elevated blood triglycerides can contribute to pancreatitis.

Gastrointestinal Cancers:

The causes of gastrointestinal cancers vary depending on the specific type and can include genetic factors, lifestyle choices (e.g., smoking, alcohol consumption), diet, infections (e.g., H. pylori in stomach cancer), and other environmental factors.

It's important to note that while these are potential causes, the exact cause of digestive problems can vary from person to person, and multiple factors may contribute to the development of these conditions. A healthcare professional can help determine the specific cause through proper evaluation and diagnostic tests.

THE CONNECTION BETWEEN DIET AND GUT HEALTH.

The connection between diet and gut health is a fundamental and intricate one. What you eat can profoundly influence the composition and activity of the gut microbiome, which in turn has a substantial impact on your overall health and well-being.

Here are some key aspects of the relationship between diet and gut health:

• Diet Shapes the Gut Microbiome: The gut microbiome is highly responsive to the foods you consume. Different types of dietary fibers, nutrients, and compounds from your diet serve as "fuel" for various microorganisms in the gut. A diverse diet rich in plant-based foods provides a wide array of nutrients that can support a balanced and diverse gut microbiome.

• Fiber and Gut Health: Dietary fiber is a key player in promoting gut health. Soluble and insoluble fibers are found in fruits, vegetables, whole grains, and legumes, and they cannot be digested by the human body. Instead, they reach the colon, where they are fermented by gut bacteria, producing short-chain fatty acids (SCFAs) that nourish the colon lining and help maintain a healthy gut environment.

• Prebiotics and Probiotics: Prebiotics are non-digestible compounds found in certain foods (e.g., garlic, onions, bananas) that serve as "food" for beneficial gut bacteria. Probiotics, on the other hand, are live microorganisms found in foods like yogurt and fermented products that can introduce beneficial bacteria to the gut. Consuming both prebiotics and probiotics can support gut health.

• Dietary Patterns: Certain dietary patterns, such as the Mediterranean diet, which is rich in fruits, vegetables, whole grains, and healthy fats, have been associated with a more diverse and beneficial gut microbiome. In contrast, diets high in processed foods, saturated fats, and added sugars are linked to less diverse and potentially less healthy gut microbiomes.

• Influence on Inflammation: Diet can modulate inflammation in the gut. A diet high in anti-inflammatory foods, such as fatty fish, nuts, and berries, can help reduce gut inflammation. Conversely, a diet high in processed and sugary foods can promote inflammation, potentially leading to gastrointestinal issues.

• Impact on Gastrointestinal Conditions: Diet can significantly affect common gastrointestinal conditions. For example, in individuals with irritable bowel syndrome (IBS), specific dietary triggers may exacerbate symptoms. In celiac disease, the elimination of gluten from the diet is essential to manage the condition.

• Weight and Metabolism: The gut microbiome plays a role in weight regulation and metabolism. A diet high in fiber and whole foods can promote satiety and support weight management. Imbalances in the gut microbiome due to a poor diet may contribute to obesity and metabolic disorders.

• Food Intolerances and Allergies: Dietary choices are crucial for individuals with food intolerances and allergies. Avoiding specific foods is essential for managing conditions like lactose intolerance, celiac disease, and various food allergies.

• Mental Health: Emerging research suggests a connection between diet, gut health, and mental health. The gut-brain axis, a bidirectional communication system between the gut and the brain, may influence mood and cognitive function. Diets rich in certain nutrients, such as omega-3 fatty acids and antioxidants, are associated with improved mental well-being.

In summary, diet is a powerful and modifiable factor that can shape the composition and function of the gut microbiome, impact gut health, and influence overall well-being. A balanced and diverse diet, rich in fiber and nutrient-dense foods, is often associated with a healthier gut microbiome and a reduced risk of gastrointestinal issues and other health conditions. If you have specific dietary concerns or are looking to optimize your gut health, it's advisable to consult with a healthcare professional or registered dietitian who can provide personalized guidance and recommendations.

GUT-FRIENDLY FOODS, FIBER, PROBIOTICS, AND PREBIOTICS.

Gut-Friendly Foods:

Gut-friendly foods are those that promote a healthy gut microbiome, support digestion, and reduce the risk of gastrointestinal issues. These foods often contain essential nutrients and compounds that nourish beneficial gut bacteria and maintain a balanced gut environment. Some examples of gut-friendly foods include:

• Fruits and Vegetables: Rich in fiber, antioxidants, and vitamins, fruits and vegetables are key components of a gut-friendly diet. They provide prebiotics and support overall gut health. Include a variety of colorful fruits and vegetables in your diet.

• Whole Grains: Whole grains like oats, brown rice, quinoa, and whole wheat are excellent sources of dietary fiber. They provide sustained energy and promote regular bowel movements.

• Legumes: Beans, lentils, and chickpeas are high in fiber and protein. They also contain prebiotics that feed beneficial gut bacteria. Incorporating legumes into your diet can support gut health.

• Yogurt: Plain, unsweetened yogurt is a source of probiotics, specifically lactic acid bacteria. It can help maintain a healthy gut microbiome by introducing beneficial bacteria.

• Fermented Foods: Foods like kefir, kimchi, sauerkraut, and kombucha are rich in live probiotics. They can help balance the gut microbiome and support digestion.

• Nuts and Seeds: Almonds, chia seeds, flaxseeds, and walnuts provide healthy fats, fiber, and other nutrients that promote gut health.

• Lean Proteins: Lean sources of protein, such as poultry, fish, and tofu, are easier to digest and contribute to overall nutrition.

• Herbs and Spices: Ginger, turmeric, and garlic have anti-inflammatory and digestive properties. They can be incorporated into meals to support gut health.

Fiber:

Dietary fiber is a type of carbohydrate found in plant-based foods that cannot be digested by the human body. Instead, it reaches the colon largely intact, where it serves as a valuable nutrient for the gut microbiome. There are two main types of dietary fiber:

• Soluble Fiber: This type of fiber dissolves in water to form a gel-like substance. It can help lower cholesterol levels and stabilize blood sugar. Soluble fiber sources include oats, beans, apples, and citrus fruits.

• Insoluble Fiber: Insoluble fiber adds bulk to the stool, facilitating regular bowel movements and preventing constipation. Sources include whole grains, nuts, and vegetables like broccoli and Brussels sprouts.

Probiotics:

Probiotics are live microorganisms that, when consumed in adequate amounts, offer health benefits. They are often referred to as "good" or "friendly" bacteria and play a crucial role in maintaining a balanced gut microbiome. Probiotic-rich foods and supplements can introduce these beneficial microorganisms into your gut. Common probiotic strains include:

• Lactobacillus: Found in yogurt, kefir, and fermented vegetables, Lactobacillus strains can help maintain gut health and support digestion.

• Bifidobacterium: Bifidobacterium strains are often used in probiotic supplements and are associated with various health benefits, including supporting a balanced gut microbiome.

• Saccharomyces boulardii: This yeast-based probiotic can be helpful in managing certain gastrointestinal conditions and preventing antibiotic-associated diarrhea.

Prebiotics:

Prebiotics are non-digestible compounds found in certain foods that serve as a food source for beneficial gut bacteria, promoting their growth and activity. Prebiotics include:

• Inulin: Found in foods like chicory root, garlic, and onions, inulin is a common prebiotic that promotes the growth of beneficial gut bacteria.

• Fructo-oligosaccharides (FOS): These compounds, present in fruits like bananas and vegetables like asparagus, provide nourishment for probiotic bacteria.

• Galacto-oligosaccharides (GOS): GOS can be found in legumes, particularly lentils and chickpeas, and are known to support the growth of beneficial gut bacteria.

• Resistant Starch: Foods like green bananas, raw potatoes, and certain grains contain resistant starch, which can serve as a prebiotic.

Including a variety of gut-friendly foods, fiber-rich sources, probiotics, and prebiotics in your diet can help support a balanced and healthy gut microbiome, maintain regular digestion, and promote overall gut health. It's important to consult with a healthcare professional or registered dietitian for personalized recommendations and guidance, especially if you have specific dietary needs or concerns.

To promote better gut health, it's important to be mindful of the foods you consume. Some foods can disrupt the balance of your gut microbiome, lead to inflammation, and contribute to gastrointestinal problems. Here are foods to avoid or limit for better gut health:

• Highly Processed Foods: Processed foods often contain additives, preservatives, and artificial ingredients that can negatively impact the gut. These items may also lack dietary fiber and beneficial nutrients. Limit foods like sugary snacks, fast food, and heavily processed convenience meals.

• Added Sugars: Excessive sugar intake can lead to imbalances in the gut microbiome and promote the growth of harmful bacteria. Sugary beverages, candies, and sweetened cereals are examples of high-sugar foods to reduce.

• Artificial Sweeteners: Some artificial sweeteners, such as saccharin and aspartame, can negatively affect gut bacteria and metabolism. It's advisable to moderate their use.

• Highly Refined Grains: Refined grains like white bread, white rice, and pasta have had their fiber-rich bran and nutrient-packed germ removed. These grains can lead to rapid spikes in blood sugar and have a negative impact on gut health.

• Saturated and Trans Fats: High intake of saturated fats (found in red meat, full-fat dairy, and fried foods) and trans fats (found in many processed and fried foods) can promote inflammation and adversely affect gut health. Opt for healthier fat sources like olive oil, avocados, and nuts.

• Red Meat: Consumption of red meat, especially processed meats like sausages and bacon, has been associated with an increased risk of certain gastrointestinal cancers. While red meat can be included in moderation, it's a good idea to limit processed meat.

• Alcohol: Excessive alcohol consumption can disrupt the gut microbiome, promote inflammation, and damage the gut lining. Limiting alcohol intake is essential for gut health.

• Artificial Additives and Preservatives: Some food additives and preservatives can negatively affect gut bacteria. Reading food labels and avoiding products with artificial additives can be beneficial.

• Highly Spiced Foods: While some spices like ginger and turmeric have anti-inflammatory properties, highly spiced foods can irritate the gut lining and lead to digestive discomfort in some individuals. Be cautious if you have a sensitive stomach.

• Dietary Triggers for Individuals: Certain foods can trigger digestive symptoms in individuals with specific sensitivities or conditions. For instance, those with lactose intolerance should avoid dairy products containing lactose. People with celiac disease must strictly avoid gluten-containing foods.

• Excessive Antibiotics and Non-Essential Medications: Overuse or unnecessary use of antibiotics can disrupt the gut microbiome. It's important to follow medical advice when taking antibiotics and other medications to minimize their impact on gut health.

• Dietary Habits That Lead to Overeating: Overeating can strain the digestive system, potentially leading to indigestion, bloating, and discomfort. It's important to practice mindful eating and portion control.

While limiting these foods can promote better gut health, it's equally important to maintain a well-rounded and diverse diet rich in fiber, whole foods, and gut-friendly items. Every individual's dietary needs and tolerances may vary, so personalized guidance from a healthcare professional or registered dietitian can help you make informed dietary choices that suit your specific circumstances.

LIFESTYLE FACTORS THAT IMPACTS GUT HEALTH

Gut health is not solely determined by diet; lifestyle factors play a significant role in shaping the gut microbiome and overall gastrointestinal well-being. Here are several lifestyle factors that can impact gut health:

• Physical Activity: Regular physical activity is associated with a more diverse and balanced gut microbiome. Exercise can help maintain healthy gut bacteria and reduce inflammation. Aim for at least 150 minutes of moderate-intensity aerobic activity per week.

• Stress Management: Chronic stress can negatively affect the gut, leading to imbalances in the microbiome and digestive problems. Practices such as meditation, deep breathing, and yoga can help manage stress and promote gut health.

• Sleep: Poor sleep patterns and insufficient sleep can disrupt the gut microbiome and increase the risk of gastrointestinal issues. Aim for 7-9 hours of quality sleep each night to support gut health.

• Hydration: Proper hydration is essential for digestion. Insufficient fluid intake can lead to constipation and affect the gut's ability to function optimally. Drinking an adequate amount of water is vital for overall gut health.

• Tobacco and Alcohol Use: Smoking and excessive alcohol consumption can disrupt the gut microbiome and contribute to digestive issues. Reducing or quitting these habits can have a positive impact on gut health.

• Medications: Certain medications, such as antibiotics, can disrupt the gut microbiome by killing both harmful and beneficial bacteria. If possible, work with your healthcare provider to minimize unnecessary use of such medications and follow their advice on maintaining gut health during treatment.

• Antibiotic Use: Antibiotics can be necessary for treating infections, but they can also disrupt the gut microbiome. If you need antibiotics, be sure to complete the full course as prescribed, and consider using probiotics during and after treatment to help restore gut balance.

• Oral Health: Poor oral hygiene and gum disease can lead to oral bacteria entering the digestive system, potentially impacting gut health. Maintain good oral hygiene practices and regular dental check-ups.

• Environmental Exposures: Exposure to environmental toxins, pollutants, and chemicals can affect the gut microbiome. Minimize exposure when possible, such as by consuming organic foods and reducing contact with harmful substances.

• Travel and Jet Lag: Changes in time zones, altered eating patterns, and exposure to new foods while traveling can temporarily affect gut health. Maintain a balanced diet, stay hydrated, and allow your digestive system to adjust to changes gradually.

• Hand Hygiene: Practicing good hand hygiene is essential to prevent the transmission of harmful pathogens to the gut. Wash your hands regularly to reduce the risk of infections.

• Social Connections: Social interactions and maintaining a strong support network can have a positive influence on mental well-being. As the gut and brain are interconnected, emotional health and social connections can indirectly affect gut health.

• Shift Work: Irregular work schedules and shift work can disrupt the body's internal clock and potentially affect gut health. Establishing regular eating and sleeping patterns can help mitigate these effects.

• Chronic Health Conditions: Certain chronic health conditions, such as diabetes and autoimmune diseases, can impact the gut microbiome. Properly managing these conditions with medical guidance can support gut health.

It's essential to adopt a holistic approach to maintaining gut health by considering both dietary and lifestyle factors. Making positive lifestyle changes, such as managing stress, getting regular exercise, and prioritizing sleep, can significantly benefit your gut and overall well-being. Consulting with a healthcare provider or registered dietitian can help you create a personalized plan for optimizing your gut health based on your specific lifestyle and health needs.

ADVICE ON HOW TO MANAGE AND IMPROVE THESE FACTORS.

Here's practical advice on how to manage and improve the lifestyle factors that impact gut health:

Physical Activity:

• Aim for at least 150 minutes of moderate-intensity aerobic exercise per week. Activities like brisk walking, swimming, or cycling can help.

• Incorporate strength training exercises to build muscle, which can further benefit gut health.

• Find activities you enjoy to make exercise a regular part of your routine. Joining a fitness class or engaging in a team sport can be motivating.

• Practice stress-reduction techniques like meditation, deep breathing exercises, or progressive muscle relaxation.

• Engage in activities you find relaxing, such as yoga, tai chi, or mindfulness.

• Maintain a healthy work-life balance and prioritize self-care.

Sleep:

• Create a sleep-conducive environment by keeping your bedroom dark, quiet, and cool.

• Establish a regular sleep schedule by going to bed and waking up at the same times every day, even on weekends.

• Limit exposure to screens (e.g., smartphones, computers, TVs) before bedtime, as the blue light can disrupt sleep.

Hydration:

• Drink an adequate amount of water throughout the day. The "8x8" rule (eight 8-ounce glasses of water per day) is a general guideline, but individual needs vary.

• Monitor your urine color; pale yellow indicates proper hydration.

Tobacco and Alcohol Use:

• Seek support and resources to quit smoking if you are a smoker.

• If you consume alcohol, do so in moderation. For example, limit alcohol to one drink per day for women and two drinks per day for men.

Medications: Only take prescribed medications as directed by your healthcare provider. Don't skip or stop medications without consulting your healthcare professional.

Antibiotic Use:

• If you need antibiotics, complete the full course as prescribed to effectively treat infections.

• Consider taking probiotics during and after antibiotic treatment to help restore the gut microbiome.

Oral Health:

• Brush and floss your teeth regularly to maintain good oral hygiene.

• Schedule regular dental check-ups and cleanings with your dentist.

Environmental Exposures:

• Choose organic foods when possible to reduce exposure to pesticides and chemicals.

• Minimize exposure to toxins and pollutants by following safety guidelines and using protective gear when needed.

Travel and Jet Lag:

• Gradually adjust your eating and sleeping patterns to the local time zone when traveling.

• Stay hydrated during flights, as airplane cabins can be dehydrating.

Hand Hygiene:

• Wash your hands regularly with soap and warm water, especially before eating or preparing food.

• Use hand sanitizer when soap and water are not available.

Social Connections:

• Foster and maintain strong social connections with friends and family.

• Engage in activities and hobbies that promote social interaction.

Shift Work:

• Establish a consistent daily routine for eating, sleeping, and exercise, even if you work irregular hours.

• Use blackout curtains to create a dark sleep environment during daylight hours.

Chronic Health Conditions:

• Work closely with your healthcare provider to manage chronic conditions effectively.

• Follow prescribed treatment plans and medications as recommended.

Remember that small, gradual changes in your lifestyle can have a positive impact on gut health over time. Building healthy habits, seeking support when needed, and making choices that prioritize your well-being are key to maintaining and improving gut health. Consulting with healthcare professionals or specialists, such as dietitians, can provide personalized guidance and recommendations for your specific health needs and goals.

A STEP-BY-STEP GUT RECOVERY PLAN THAT INCLUDES DIETARY RECOMMENDATIONS AND MEAL PLANS

Creating a gut recovery plan involves making gradual and sustainable changes to your diet and lifestyle. Here's a step-by-step guide, including dietary recommendations and sample meal plans to help you get started on your journey to better gut health:

Step 1: Assess Your Current Diet and Lifestyle

Before making changes, assess your current diet, lifestyle, and any digestive issues you're experiencing. Consider keeping a food diary to track your eating habits.

Step 2: Set Clear Goals

Determine your specific gut health goals, such as reducing bloating, improving regularity, or managing digestive discomfort. Having clear goals will guide your plan.

Step 3: Dietary Recommendations

Phase 1: Elimination and Reset (2-4 Weeks)

Foods to Avoid:

• Highly processed foods

• Added sugars and artificial sweeteners

• Refined grains

• Saturated and trans fats

• Excessive red and processed meats

• Alcohol

Foods to Focus On:

• Whole, unprocessed foods

• Fiber-rich fruits and vegetables

• Whole grains

• Legumes

• Lean proteins (poultry, fish, tofu)

• Healthy fats (olive oil, avocados, nuts)

• Probiotic-rich foods (plain yogurt, kefir, fermented vegetables)

Sample Phase 1 Meal Plan:

Breakfast:

• Greek yogurt with mixed berries and a drizzle of honey.

• Whole-grain toast with almond butter.

Lunch:

• Grilled chicken breast salad with mixed greens, cherry tomatoes, and balsamic vinaigrette.

• A serving of quinoa.

Snack:

• Sliced cucumbers and carrots with hummus.

Dinner:

• Baked salmon with lemon and dill.

• Steamed broccoli and brown rice.

Phase 2: Gut-Friendly Foods (Ongoing)

In this phase, continue to avoid processed and sugary foods while introducing more gut-friendly options.

Foods to Add:

• Prebiotic-rich foods (garlic, onions, bananas, asparagus)

• Fermented foods (kimchi, sauerkraut, kefir)

• Herbs and spices with gut benefits (ginger, turmeric)

Sample Phase 2 Meal Plan:

Breakfast:

• Oatmeal topped with sliced banana and a sprinkle of chia seeds.

• A cup of green tea.

Lunch:

• Lentil and vegetable soup.

• Mixed greens salad with vinaigrette dressing.

Snack:

• A small serving of kefir or a piece of dark chocolate.

Dinner:

• Stir-fried tofu with broccoli, bell peppers, and a ginger-turmeric sauce.

• Quinoa or brown rice.

Step 4: Lifestyle Changes

• Prioritize stress management techniques such as meditation, yoga, or deep breathing exercises.

• Maintain regular physical activity, aiming for at least 150 minutes of moderate-intensity exercise each week.

• Ensure you get 7-9 hours of quality sleep per night.

• Maintain proper hydration throughout the day.

• Limit alcohol consumption and quit smoking if you are a smoker.

• Practice good hand hygiene and maintain oral health.

Step 5: Monitor and Adjust

• Keep a food diary and note any changes in your digestive symptoms, energy levels, and overall well-being.

• Gradually reintroduce some previously eliminated foods to assess how your gut responds.

• Consult with a registered dietitian or healthcare professional for guidance and personalized recommendations based on your specific needs.

Remember that gut health is highly individual, and what works for one person may not work for another. Be patient with yourself, and make adjustments based on your own experience and progress. The key is to create a sustainable gut recovery plan that promotes long-term health and well-being.

Supplements and probiotics can be valuable additions to your gut health regimen when used thoughtfully and with guidance from a healthcare professional. Here's detailed information on supplements and probiotics:

1. Probiotics:

Probiotics are live microorganisms that, when taken in adequate amounts, can provide various health benefits, particularly for gut health. They help maintain a balanced and diverse gut microbiome. There are numerous strains of probiotics, and each may have unique effects. Here's what you should know:

• Common Probiotic Strains: Some well-known probiotic strains include Lactobacillus acidophilus, Bifidobacterium bifidum, and Saccharomyces boulardii. These strains can help with conditions like diarrhea, irritable bowel syndrome (IBS), and maintaining gut balance.

• Conditions Benefitted: Probiotics are often used to manage gastrointestinal conditions such as diarrhea (including antibiotic-associated diarrhea), constipation, and IBS. They may also support gut health in individuals with inflammatory bowel disease (IBD) or when taking antibiotics.

• Forms: Probiotics are available in various forms, including capsules, powders, and liquid supplements. They are also found in certain foods, such as yogurt, kefir, and fermented vegetables.

• Dosage: The appropriate dosage can vary depending on the probiotic strain and the specific condition you are addressing. Follow the recommended dosage on the product label, and consider consulting a healthcare professional for guidance.

• Timing: Probiotics can be taken with or without food, but consistency in timing is important. Some people find it helpful to take them with a meal to minimize stomach upset.

• Side Effects: Probiotics are generally safe, but some people may experience mild side effects such as gas, bloating, or an upset stomach when they first start taking them. These symptoms usually subside as your body adjusts.

• Storage: Store probiotics according to the manufacturer's instructions, usually in a cool, dry place, and be mindful of their expiration dates.

2. Prebiotics:

Prebiotics are non-digestible compounds found in certain foods that serve as a food source for beneficial gut bacteria, promoting their growth and activity. They help create a healthy environment for probiotics to thrive. Common prebiotics include inulin, fructo-oligosaccharides (FOS), and galacto-oligosaccharides (GOS). Prebiotic-rich foods include garlic, onions, asparagus, bananas, and whole grains.

3. Fiber Supplements:

Dietary fiber is essential for gut health, as it helps maintain regular bowel movements and supports a healthy gut microbiome. If your diet is low in fiber, you may consider fiber supplements. Psyllium husk and wheat dextrin are common sources of soluble fiber, while methylcellulose and calcium polycarbophil are examples of bulk-forming fiber supplements.

4. Digestive Enzymes:

Digestive enzyme supplements can be helpful for individuals with conditions that affect their ability to digest and absorb nutrients properly, such as pancreatic insufficiency. These supplements contain enzymes like amylase, protease, and lipase, which aid in the breakdown of carbohydrates, proteins, and fats, respectively.

5. L-Glutamine:

L-Glutamine is an amino acid that plays a role in maintaining the integrity of the intestinal lining. It may be beneficial for individuals with conditions such as leaky gut syndrome or inflammatory bowel disease.

6. Zinc Carnosine:

Zinc carnosine is a supplement that can help support gut health and protect the mucosal lining of the stomach. It's often used for individuals with conditions like gastritis or peptic ulcers.

7. Consult a Healthcare Professional:

It's crucial to consult a healthcare professional before starting any new supplements, especially if you have underlying health conditions or are taking medications. They can help determine which supplements are appropriate for your specific needs and provide guidance on dosage and safety.

Remember that supplements should complement a well-balanced diet and a healthy lifestyle, not replace them. A holistic approach to gut health, which includes a fiber-rich diet, probiotics, and lifestyle modifications, is often the most effective way to promote long-term gut well-being.

ADDITIONAL TIPS AND STRATEGIES FOR MAINTAINING LONG-TERM GUT HEALTH.

Maintaining long-term gut health requires consistent, sustainable practices. Here are additional tips and strategies to support your gut health over the long term:

1. Eat a Diverse Diet:

Consume a wide variety of fruits, vegetables, whole grains, and legumes. Different foods provide different nutrients and fibers that nourish various beneficial gut bacteria.

2. Practice Mindful Eating:

Eat slowly, savor your food, and pay attention to your body's hunger and fullness cues. Mindful eating can help reduce overeating and promote healthy digestion.

3. Stay Hydrated:

Drink an adequate amount of water throughout the day to support digestive processes and help prevent constipation.

4. Limit Antibiotic Use:

Use antibiotics only when necessary and as prescribed by a healthcare professional. Overuse of antibiotics can disrupt the gut microbiome.

5. Avoid Overuse of Pain Medications:

Limit the use of nonsteroidal anti-inflammatory drugs (NSAIDs) like aspirin and ibuprofen, which can irritate the stomach lining and lead to gastrointestinal problems.

6. Limit Alcohol and Tobacco:

Moderate alcohol consumption and, if possible, quit smoking. Both alcohol and tobacco can negatively impact gut health.

7. Manage Stress:

Incorporate stress-reduction techniques like meditation, yoga, or deep breathing exercises into your daily routine. Chronic stress can disrupt the gut microbiome.

8. Stay Physically Active:

Engage in regular physical activity, such as walking, jogging, or strength training, to promote gut health. Exercise can support the balance of gut bacteria and reduce inflammation.

9. Prioritize Sleep:

Aim for 7-9 hours of quality sleep each night. Proper sleep patterns help maintain a healthy gut microbiome.

10. Oral Hygiene:

Maintain good oral hygiene practices, such as brushing and flossing your teeth regularly. Poor oral health can affect gut health when oral bacteria enter the digestive system.

11. Regular Check-ups:

Schedule regular health check-ups with your healthcare provider. Discuss any digestive symptoms or concerns you may have.

12. Fiber Maintenance:

Continue to consume a diet rich in fiber to support regular bowel movements and gut health. Whole foods are the best sources of dietary fiber.

13. Keep a Food Diary:

Periodically assess your dietary habits and gut health symptoms by keeping a food diary. Note any foods that seem to trigger discomfort or symptoms.

14. Avoid Excessive Antibiotics:

If possible, work with your healthcare provider to avoid overusing antibiotics. In some cases, alternatives or narrower-spectrum antibiotics may be considered.

15. Reduce Environmental Toxins:

Minimize exposure to environmental toxins and pollutants that can negatively affect the gut microbiome.

16. Social Connections:

Foster and maintain social connections and engage in activities that promote social interaction. Emotional well-being indirectly affects gut health.

17. Herbs and Spices:

Incorporate gut-friendly herbs and spices like ginger, turmeric, and garlic into your meals to support digestion and reduce inflammation.

18. Consult with Healthcare Professionals:

If you have specific gut health concerns or conditions, consult with a healthcare provider, registered dietitian, or gastroenterologist for personalized advice and guidance.

Maintaining long-term gut health is a holistic journey that involves a balanced diet, lifestyle choices, and an awareness of how your body responds to different foods and stressors. Consistency and a mindful approach to your gut health practices will contribute to your overall well-being over time.

Reintroducing certain foods after an elimination or reset phase can be a valuable step in assessing your gut's response to different dietary components. Here's some advice on how to reintroduce foods and effectively track your progress:

1. Start Gradually:

Begin with one food at a time. This helps you pinpoint which specific foods may trigger digestive symptoms or discomfort.

2. Choose High-Quality Foods:

Opt for whole and minimally processed versions of the food you're reintroducing. This will help ensure that the food itself is the focus, rather than additives or preservatives.

3. Keep a Food Diary:

Create a food diary to track your reintroductions. Include details like the date, the specific food, portion size, and any immediate or delayed symptoms (e.g., bloating, gas, diarrhea).

4. Observe Symptoms:

Pay close attention to your body's response to the reintroduced food. Some reactions may occur immediately, while others could be delayed by several hours or even a day.

5. Wait for Several Days:

Monitor your symptoms for at least a few days (up to a week) after reintroducing the food. This extended observation period is essential because some digestive issues may not surface immediately.

6. Rate Your Comfort Levels:

Use a scale, such as 1 to 5, to rate how comfortable or uncomfortable you feel after eating the reintroduced food. This can help you quantify and track your symptoms.

7. Rotate Foods:

Introduce one food at a time and, if there are no symptoms or discomfort, rotate it with other foods in your diet to ensure you're not consuming it too frequently.

8. Gradually Increase Portions:

If you tolerate the reintroduced food without issues, gradually increase the portion size over several days to see if your gut can handle larger amounts.

9. Be Patient:

The process of reintroducing foods can be slow, and it's essential to be patient and methodical. Rushing this process can make it challenging to identify specific triggers.

10. Record Reactions:

Document any reactions or symptoms you experience for each food you reintroduce. This information will be helpful in determining which foods you can tolerate and which you should continue to avoid.

11. Seek Professional Guidance:

If you have a history of severe food allergies, intolerances, or gastrointestinal conditions, or if you are unsure how to reintroduce certain foods, consult with a healthcare professional, registered dietitian, or gastroenterologist. They can provide guidance, allergy testing, or specialized reintroduction protocols.

12. Personalize Your Approach:

Your gut health is unique, and what triggers symptoms in one person may not affect another. Personalize your approach based on your specific sensitivities and dietary goals.

13. Be Open to Adjustments:

As you reintroduce foods, be prepared to make adjustments to your diet based on your body's responses. You may need to continue avoiding specific foods or find alternatives that are better tolerated.

14. Listen to Your Body:

Ultimately, trust your body's signals. If a particular food consistently causes digestive discomfort or symptoms, it may be best to limit or avoid it in the long term.

Reintroducing foods can be a valuable tool for fine-tuning your diet, but it's essential to approach the process systematically and patiently. By keeping a detailed food diary, observing your body's reactions, and seeking professional guidance if necessary, you can make informed decisions about which foods to include or exclude from your diet for the sake of your gut health.

Consulting a healthcare professional for gut issues is of paramount importance for several reasons:

1. Accurate Diagnosis: Healthcare professionals, particularly gastroenterologists, are trained to diagnose and differentiate various gut-related conditions. They can perform tests, screenings, and evaluations to identify the underlying cause of your symptoms. Accurate diagnosis is the first step in effective treatment.

2. Tailored Treatment Plans: Once a diagnosis is made, healthcare professionals can create personalized treatment plans that address the specific gut issue you're facing. These plans take into account your medical history, current health, and individual needs.

3. Medication Management: For certain gastrointestinal conditions, medications may be necessary to manage symptoms and promote healing. Healthcare professionals can prescribe and monitor the use of medications to ensure safety and efficacy.

4. Preventive Measures: Healthcare professionals can provide guidance on preventive measures, lifestyle changes, and dietary modifications to reduce the risk of future gut issues and promote long-term gut health.

5. Expert Knowledge: Gastrointestinal health is a specialized field, and healthcare professionals have in-depth knowledge of the digestive system and its intricacies. This expertise enables them to provide the most accurate and up-to-date information and advice.

6. Monitoring Progress: For chronic gut issues, regular follow-up visits with a healthcare professional are crucial to monitor your progress and make necessary adjustments to your treatment plan. They can assess whether your condition is improving or if changes are needed.

7. Treatment of Complex Conditions: Some gut issues, such as inflammatory bowel disease (IBD), celiac disease, and gastrointestinal cancers, can be complex and require specialized care. Healthcare professionals are equipped to manage these conditions effectively.

8. Diagnostic Procedures: Healthcare professionals have access to a range of diagnostic procedures, such as endoscopy, colonoscopy, and imaging tests, to visualize and assess the gut's condition and functionality.

9. Identifying Red Flags: Some gut issues can be symptoms of more severe medical conditions. Healthcare professionals are trained to recognize red flags and potential warning signs that may require further investigation.

10. Emotional Support: Dealing with chronic gut issues can be emotionally challenging. Healthcare professionals can offer emotional support and connect you with resources and support groups for coping with the psychological aspects of gut health.

11. Avoiding Misdiagnosis and Self-Medication: Self-diagnosis and self-medication can lead to inaccurate conclusions and may exacerbate the problem. A healthcare professional can help you

avoid potential misdiagnoses and provide evidence-based treatment.

12. Preventing Complications: Timely intervention and treatment under the guidance of a healthcare professional can help prevent complications, improve quality of life, and reduce the risk of long-term health issues.

In conclusion, consulting a healthcare professional for gut issues is essential for obtaining an accurate diagnosis, receiving appropriate treatment, and ensuring the best possible outcome for your gut health. Their expertise and guidance can lead to a more accurate understanding of your condition and more effective management of gut-related concerns.

STRESS REDUCTION TECHNIQUES AND ITS IMPACT ON GUT HEALTH

Stress reduction techniques have a significant impact on gut health, as the gut and brain are intricately connected through the gut-brain axis. Chronic stress can lead to adverse effects on the gastrointestinal system and disrupt the balance of the gut microbiome. Here are some stress reduction techniques and their positive impact on gut health:

1. Mindfulness Meditation:

Mindfulness meditation involves focusing on the present moment and accepting it without judgment. Regular practice can reduce the production of stress hormones and alleviate symptoms of gastrointestinal disorders.

2. Deep Breathing Exercises:

Deep, slow breathing techniques, such as diaphragmatic breathing, activate the body's relaxation response, promoting digestion and reducing stress-related gut symptoms.

3. Progressive Muscle Relaxation:

Progressive muscle relaxation involves tensing and relaxing muscle groups in the body. It can help relieve muscle tension and reduce stress, which may benefit gut health.

4. Yoga:

Yoga combines physical postures, breathing exercises, and meditation to promote relaxation and reduce stress. It has been shown to improve symptoms in individuals with IBS and other gut disorders.

5. Tai Chi:

Tai Chi is a mind-body practice that combines gentle movements and deep breathing. Regular practice can reduce stress, improve gut motility, and alleviate digestive symptoms.

6. Aerobic Exercise:

Engaging in regular aerobic exercise can reduce stress and promote the release of endorphins, which can positively impact gut health and maintain a balanced gut microbiome.

7. Sleep Hygiene:

Ensuring you get 7-9 hours of quality sleep each night is essential for managing stress and promoting gut health. Poor sleep patterns can disrupt the gut microbiome and lead to gastrointestinal issues.

8. Cognitive Behavioral Therapy (CBT):

CBT is a type of psychotherapy that helps individuals identify and manage stressors and negative thought patterns. It can be effective in reducing stress-related gut symptoms.

9. Social Support:

Maintaining a strong support network of friends and family can provide emotional and psychological support, which can indirectly impact gut health by reducing stress levels.

10. Time Management:

Efficient time management and organization can help reduce stress associated with work and daily responsibilities, leading to improved gut health.

11. Biofeedback:

Biofeedback techniques can help individuals gain control over physical processes that are typically involuntary, such as heart rate and muscle tension, leading to reduced stress and improved gut function.

12. Adequate Hydration:

Staying properly hydrated can help maintain physiological functions, reduce stress, and support gut health.

The impact of stress on gut health is well-documented, and these techniques can help mitigate the negative effects. Reducing stress through these methods may lead to improved gastrointestinal comfort, reduced inflammation, and a healthier gut microbiome. However, it's essential to choose stress reduction techniques that work best for you and incorporate them into your daily routine to achieve long-lasting benefits for both your mental and gut health.

TYPES OF EXERCISES TO HELP MAINTAIN A HEALTHY GUT

Exercise plays a crucial role in maintaining a healthy gut, as it can positively influence gut motility, the gut microbiome, and overall digestive well-being. Here are some types of exercises that can support gut health:

1. Aerobic Exercises:

Aerobic exercises, such as brisk walking, jogging, cycling, and swimming, can stimulate gut motility and promote regular bowel movements. These activities increase blood flow to the digestive organs, aiding in digestion.

2. Yoga:

Yoga combines physical postures, controlled breathing, and meditation. It can help reduce stress, which is known to impact gut health. Certain yoga poses, like twists and stretches, can also target the abdominal area, aiding digestion.

3. Tai Chi:

Tai Chi is a low-impact exercise that incorporates slow, flowing movements and deep breathing. It can help reduce stress and improve gut motility.

4. Pilates:

Pilates exercises focus on core strength, flexibility, and posture. Strengthening the core muscles can indirectly support digestive health by improving abdominal muscle function.

5. High-Intensity Interval Training (HIIT):

HIIT involves short bursts of intense exercise followed by brief rest periods. It can boost metabolism, improve cardiovascular health, and indirectly benefit gut health.

6. Strength Training:

Resistance training, such as weight lifting or bodyweight exercises, helps build muscle and increase overall metabolism. A well-functioning metabolism can promote efficient digestion and nutrient absorption.

7. Bodyweight Exercises:

Bodyweight exercises like squats, lunges, and planks can help improve core strength and overall fitness, which can support gut health.

8. Outdoor Activities:

Exercising in natural settings, such as hiking or trail running, can have added benefits for gut health by exposing you to diverse environments and microorganisms.

9. Gentle Stretching:

Gentle stretching exercises, like those in a stretching routine or during a restorative yoga class, can relieve muscle tension, which may indirectly reduce stress and benefit gut function.

10. Belly Breathing:

Deep belly breathing exercises help relax the body and activate the parasympathetic nervous system, which can improve digestion and reduce stress.

11. Swimming:

Swimming is a full-body exercise that can promote overall fitness and reduce stress, potentially benefiting gut health.

12. Hiking and Nature Walks:

Spending time in nature, hiking, or taking long walks can help reduce stress and support mental well-being, which in turn can positively influence gut health.

It's important to choose exercises that you enjoy and can incorporate into your regular routine. Consistency is key for maintaining gut health, so aim for a balanced exercise regimen that includes both aerobic and strength-building activities.

Additionally, staying hydrated during exercise is essential for overall well-being, including gut health. Always consult with a healthcare professional or fitness expert before starting a new exercise program, especially if you have any underlying health conditions.

IMPORTANCE OF A FOOD DIARY

A food diary, also known as a food journal or food log, is a valuable tool for various aspects of health and well-being. Here are some key reasons why maintaining a food diary is important:

1. Promotes Awareness:

Keeping a food diary encourages you to become more mindful of your eating habits. It helps you pay closer attention to what, when, and why you're eating.

2. Identifies Patterns and Triggers:

By tracking your food intake, you can identify patterns and triggers that may be affecting your health. For example, you may notice a correlation between certain foods and digestive discomfort or between emotional stress and overeating.

3. Supports Weight Management:

A food diary can be a useful tool for weight management. It helps you track your calorie intake, portion sizes, and the quality of your food choices, which can aid in achieving weight-related goals.

4. Evaluates Nutrient Intake:

It allows you to assess your daily nutrient intake, helping you ensure you're meeting your dietary requirements for vitamins, minerals, and other essential nutrients.

5. Enhances Accountability:

Knowing that you're documenting your food choices can help you make more mindful and healthier decisions. It can serve as a form of accountability to yourself.

6. Identifies Allergies and Intolerances:

Keeping a food diary can be instrumental in identifying food allergies or intolerances. If you notice a recurring pattern of symptoms after consuming specific foods, it may indicate an issue that requires further investigation.

7. Supports Dietary Goals:

Whether you're following a specific diet plan, trying to reduce sugar intake, or increasing fiber consumption, a food diary can help you track your progress and adherence to your dietary goals.

8. Assists in Digestive Health:

For individuals with digestive issues, a food diary can help pinpoint triggers for symptoms like bloating, gas, or acid reflux. This information is valuable when working with healthcare professionals to diagnose and manage gut-related conditions.

9. Encourages Informed Choices:

Reviewing your food diary can help you make informed choices about your diet. You can identify which foods make you feel your best and which ones you might want to consume in moderation or avoid.

10. Facilitates Personalization:

A food diary is a tool for personalization. It allows you to tailor your diet to your individual needs and preferences, helping you find a sustainable, long-term approach to eating.

11. Promotes Mind-Body Connection:

Keeping a food diary can deepen your awareness of the connection between what you eat and how you feel physically and emotionally, fostering a holistic view of health.

12. Encourages Accountability in Health Challenges:

If you're dealing with specific health challenges, such as diabetes, heart disease, or gastrointestinal issues, a food diary can be an essential part of your self-management plan.

Overall, a food diary is a powerful tool for self-reflection, self-improvement, and overall health and wellness. It can help you make more informed dietary choices, identify areas for improvement, and work towards your health and wellness goals, whether they relate to weight management, gut health, or general well-being.

Greek Yogurt Parfait

Ingredients:

• 1 cup Greek yogurt (unsweetened)

• 1/2 cup mixed berries (blueberries, strawberries, or raspberries)

• 1 tablespoon honey or maple syrup (optional)

• 2 tablespoons granola

• 1 tablespoon chia seeds

Instructions:

1. In a glass or bowl, start with a layer of Greek yogurt.

2. Add a layer of mixed berries on top of the yogurt. Drizzle honey or maple syrup for sweetness, if desired.

3. Sprinkle granola and chia seeds for added fiber and crunch. Repeat the layers as desired, and enjoy!

Ingredients:

- 1/2 cup old-fashioned oats

- 1 cup water or milk (dairy or non-dairy)

- 1 ripe banana, sliced

- 1 tablespoon almond butter

- 1 tablespoon chopped almonds

- Cinnamon and honey (optional, for flavor)

Instructions:

1. In a saucepan, bring water or milk to a boil.

2. Stir in the oats and reduce the heat to simmer. Cook for about 5 minutes, stirring occasionally.

3. Once the oats are creamy, remove from heat. Top the oatmeal with banana slices, almond butter, chopped almonds, and a sprinkle of cinnamon.

4. Drizzle honey if you prefer additional sweetness.

Ingredients:

• 2 eggs

• 1 cup fresh spinach, chopped

• 1/2 ripe avocado, diced

• Salt and pepper, to taste

• Olive oil for cooking

Instructions:

1. In a bowl, beat the eggs and season with salt and pepper.

2. Heat a pan over medium heat with a little olive oil. Add the chopped spinach and sauté until wilted.

3. Pour in the beaten eggs and cook, stirring gently, until they are scrambled to your liking.

4. Serve the scrambled eggs with diced avocado on top.

Whole-Grain Toast with Almond Butter and Berries

Ingredients:

• 2 slices of whole-grain bread

• 2 tablespoons almond butter

• 1/2 cup mixed berries (strawberries, blackberries, or raspberries)

Instructions:

1. Toast the slices of whole-grain bread until they're crisp.

2. Spread almond butter evenly on each slice.

3. Top with mixed berries, and press them gently into the almond butter.

Chia Seed Pudding with Mango

Ingredients:

• 2 tablespoons chia seeds

• 1/2 cup unsweetened almond milk (or any preferred milk)

• 1/2 ripe mango, diced

• 1 teaspoon honey (optional, for sweetness)

Instructions:

1. In a bowl or jar, mix the chia seeds and almond milk. Stir well to avoid clumping.

2. Cover and refrigerate for at least 3 hours or overnight until it thickens.

3. When ready to serve, top the chia pudding with diced mango.

4. Drizzle with honey for extra sweetness if desired.

Spinach and Mushroom Omelette

Ingredients:

• 2 eggs

• 1 cup fresh spinach, chopped

• 1/2 cup sliced mushrooms

• 1/4 cup diced onions

• Salt and pepper, to taste

• Olive oil for cooking

Instructions:

1. In a bowl, beat the eggs and season with salt and pepper.

2. Heat a non-stick skillet over medium heat with a little olive oil.

3. Add onions and mushrooms and sauté until they soften. Add the chopped spinach and cook until wilted.

4. Pour the beaten eggs over the vegetables and cook until the omelette is set. Fold it in half and serve.

Quinoa Breakfast Bowl

Ingredients:

• 1/2 cup cooked quinoa

• 1/4 cup Greek yogurt

• 1/2 cup mixed berries (blueberries, strawberries, or raspberries)

• 1 tablespoon honey

• 1 tablespoon chopped almonds

Instructions:

1. In a bowl, layer the cooked quinoa, Greek yogurt, and mixed berries.

2. Drizzle honey for sweetness.

3. Sprinkle chopped almonds for added texture and flavor.

Smoothie Bowl

Ingredients:

• 1 cup unsweetened yogurt (dairy or non-dairy)

• 1/2 frozen banana

• 1/2 cup mixed berries

• 1 tablespoon chia seeds

• 1/4 cup granola

• Honey or maple syrup (optional, for sweetness)

Instructions:

1. Blend the yogurt, frozen banana, and mixed berries until smooth.

2. Pour the smoothie into a bowl.

3. Top with chia seeds, granola, and drizzle with honey or maple syrup if desired.

Brown Rice Porridge with Cinnamon and Apple

Ingredients:

• 1/2 cup cooked brown rice

• 1/2 cup unsweetened almond milk

• 1/2 apple, diced

• 1/2 teaspoon ground cinnamon

• 1 tablespoon chopped walnuts (optional)

Instructions:

1. In a saucepan, combine the cooked brown rice and almond milk.

2. Heat over medium heat, stirring occasionally, until the mixture thickens. Stir in diced apples and ground cinnamon.

3. Cook until the apples soften and the porridge is creamy.

4. Top with chopped walnuts for added crunch.

Berry and Oat Breakfast Smoothie

Ingredients:

• 1/2 cup rolled oats

• 1 cup unsweetened almond milk (or any preferred milk)

• 1/2 cup mixed berries (blueberries, strawberries, or raspberries)

• 1 tablespoon honey or maple syrup (optional)

Instructions:

1. In a blender, combine rolled oats, almond milk, mixed berries, and honey (if using).

2. Blend until smooth and creamy.

3. Pour the smoothie into a glass or bowl and enjoy.

Ingredients:

• 2 tablespoons chia seeds

• 1 cup unsweetened almond milk (or any preferred milk)

• 1/2 cup mixed berries (blueberries, strawberries, or raspberries)

• 1 tablespoon honey (optional, for sweetness)

Instructions:

1. In a jar or bowl, combine chia seeds and almond milk. Mix well.

2. Add mixed berries on top and drizzle with honey for added sweetness, if desired.

3. Cover and refrigerate overnight. The chia seeds will absorb the liquid and create a pudding-like consistency.

Gut-Healthy Smoothie

Ingredients:

• 1 cup kefir (a fermented dairy product) or dairy-free alternative

• 1 ripe banana

• 1/2 cup fresh papaya

• 1 tablespoon ground flaxseeds

• A handful of baby spinach (optional)

• Honey or maple syrup (optional, for sweetness)

Instructions:

1. Blend kefir, banana, papaya, ground flaxseeds, and spinach (if using) until smooth.

2. Sweeten with honey or maple syrup, if desired.

3. Enjoy a nutrient-packed smoothie that supports gut health.

Vegetable and Herb Scramble

Ingredients:

• 2 eggs

- 1/4 cup diced bell peppers

- 1/4 cup diced tomatoes

- 2 tablespoons chopped fresh herbs (e.g., basil, parsley, chives)

- Salt and pepper, to taste

- Olive oil for cooking

Instructions:

1. Beat the eggs and season with salt and pepper. Heat a non-stick skillet with a little olive oil over medium heat.

2. Add the diced bell peppers and sauté until slightly softened. Add the tomatoes and cook for a few minutes.

3. Pour in the beaten eggs and cook, stirring occasionally, until they're scrambled.

4. Sprinkle with fresh herbs and serve.

Gut-Healthy Acai Bowl

Ingredients:

- 1 packet of frozen acai puree

- 1/2 cup unsweetened almond milk (or any preferred milk)

- 1 ripe banana

- 1/4 cup mixed berries

- Toppings: sliced banana, granola, chia seeds, honey

Instructions:

1. In a blender, combine the acai puree, almond milk, banana, and mixed berries. Blend until smooth.

2. Pour the acai mixture into a bowl.

3. Top with sliced banana, granola, chia seeds, and drizzle with honey.

Gut-Healthy Avocado Toast

Ingredients:

- 2 slices of whole-grain or sourdough bread

- 1 ripe avocado

- Cherry tomatoes, sliced

• Arugula leaves

• Lemon juice, salt, and pepper for seasoning

Instructions:

1. Toast the bread until crisp. Mash the ripe avocado and spread it evenly on the toast.

2. Top with sliced cherry tomatoes, arugula, and a drizzle of lemon juice.

3. Season with salt and pepper to taste.

Fermented Yogurt Bowl

Ingredients:

• 1 cup plain, unsweetened yogurt (Greek or regular)

• 1/2 cup sliced kiwi

• 2 tablespoons honey

• 1/4 cup mixed nuts (almonds, walnuts, or pecans)

• A pinch of ground cinnamon

Instructions:

1. In a bowl, scoop the plain yogurt.

2. Top with sliced kiwi and drizzle with honey.

3. Sprinkle mixed nuts and a pinch of ground cinnamon for added flavor and texture.

Sweet Potato and Black Bean Breakfast Burrito

Ingredients:

• 1 small cooked sweet potato, diced

• 1/2 cup canned black beans, drained and rinsed

• 2 large eggs

• Whole-grain tortilla

• Salsa or hot sauce (optional)

• Fresh cilantro, chopped (optional)

Instructions:

1. In a skillet, sauté the diced sweet potato and black beans until heated through.

2. In a separate pan, scramble the eggs. Warm the whole-grain tortilla.

3. Assemble the burrito by placing the sweet potato and black bean mixture in the tortilla, topping with scrambled eggs.

4. Add salsa or hot sauce and fresh cilantro for extra flavor.

Gut-Healthy Fruit Salad

Ingredients:

• 1 cup mixed fruit (e.g., pineapple, papaya, kiwi, and mango)

• 1/4 cup unsweetened coconut flakes

• A squeeze of fresh lime juice

• Fresh mint leaves for garnish

Instructions:

1. Dice the mixed fruit and combine them in a bowl. Sprinkle with unsweetened coconut flakes.

2. Squeeze fresh lime juice over the fruit for a zesty twist.

3. Garnish with fresh mint leaves.

Gut-Healthy Avocado and Salmon Toast

Ingredients:

• 2 slices of whole-grain or sourdough bread

• 1 ripe avocado

• Smoked salmon slices

• Red onion, thinly sliced

• Capers (optional)

• Fresh dill or chives, chopped

• Lemon juice, salt, and pepper for seasoning

Instructions:

1. Toast the bread until crisp. Mash the ripe avocado and spread it evenly on the toast.

2. Layer with smoked salmon slices, red onion, and capers if desired.

3. Sprinkle fresh dill or chives and season with lemon juice, salt, and pepper.

Ingredients:

• 1 ripe banana

• 1/2 cup rolled oats

• 1/4 cup unsweetened almond milk (or any preferred milk)

• 1 teaspoon honey or maple syrup (optional)

• Fresh berries for topping

Instructions:

1. In a blender, combine the ripe banana, rolled oats, almond milk, and honey (if using).

2. Blend until you have a smooth pancake batter.

3. Heat a non-stick pan over medium heat and pour small portions of the batter to make pancakes.

4. Cook until the edges are set and bubbles form on the surface, then flip and cook the other side.

5. Top with fresh berries and additional honey or maple syrup if desired.

Gut-Healing Quinoa Salad

Ingredients:

- 1 cup cooked quinoa

- 1 cup mixed greens (e.g., spinach, kale)

- 1/2 cup chickpeas (canned and rinsed)

- 1/4 cup diced cucumber

- 1/4 cup diced red bell pepper

- 1/4 cup cherry tomatoes, halved

- 2 tablespoons extra-virgin olive oil

- 1 tablespoon lemon juice

- 1 teaspoon ground cumin

- Salt and pepper to taste

Instructions:

1. In a large bowl, combine quinoa, mixed greens, chickpeas, cucumber, red bell pepper, and cherry tomatoes.

2. In a small bowl, whisk together olive oil, lemon juice, ground cumin, salt, and pepper.

3. Drizzle the dressing over the salad and toss to combine.

Gut-Friendly Lentil Soup

Ingredients:

• 1 cup dried green or brown lentils, rinsed

• 1 onion, diced

• 2 carrots, diced

• 2 celery stalks, diced

• 4 cups vegetable broth

• 1 teaspoon ground cumin

• 1 teaspoon ground coriander

• Salt and pepper to taste

• Fresh parsley or cilantro for garnish

Instructions:

1. In a large pot, sauté the onion, carrots, and celery until they soften.

2. Add the lentils, vegetable broth, ground cumin, and ground coriander.

3. Bring to a boil, then reduce heat and simmer for about 20-25 minutes or until the lentils are tender.

4. Season with salt and pepper. Garnish with fresh parsley or cilantro before serving.

Gut-Healthy Salmon and Quinoa Bowl

Ingredients:

• 1 cup cooked quinoa

• 4 oz salmon fillet, grilled or baked

• 1 cup steamed broccoli florets

• 1/4 cup diced red cabbage

- 1/4 cup shredded carrots

- Lemon-tahini dressing: 2 tablespoons tahini, 1 tablespoon lemon juice, and 1-2 tablespoons water to thin

- Salt and pepper to taste

Instructions:

1. Place the cooked quinoa in a bowl. Top with the grilled or baked salmon.

2. Add steamed broccoli, diced red cabbage, and shredded carrots.

3. Drizzle the lemon-tahini dressing over the bowl. Season with salt and pepper.

Gut-Healing Tofu and Vegetable Stir-Fry

Ingredients:

- 1 cup extra-firm tofu, cubed

- 2 cups mixed vegetables (e.g., bell peppers, broccoli, snap peas)

- 2 tablespoons low-sodium soy sauce or tamari

- 1 tablespoon sesame oil

- 1 teaspoon grated fresh ginger

- 2 cloves garlic, minced

- 2 cups cooked brown rice

Instructions:

1. In a wok or large pan, heat the sesame oil over medium-high heat.

2. Add the cubed tofu and cook until lightly browned. Stir in the grated ginger and minced garlic.

3. Add the mixed vegetables and cook until they're tender-crisp. Drizzle with soy sauce or tamari and stir well.

4. Serve over cooked brown rice.

Gut-Friendly Chickpea and Avocado Wrap

Ingredients:

- 1 whole-grain or gluten-free tortilla

• 1/2 cup canned chickpeas, drained and rinsed

• 1/2 ripe avocado, sliced

• 1/4 cup mixed greens (e.g., spinach, arugula)

• 1/4 cup shredded carrots

• Hummus or tahini for spreading

• Lemon juice, salt, and pepper for seasoning

Instructions:

1. Warm the tortilla in a dry skillet or microwave for a few seconds. Spread a layer of hummus or tahini on the tortilla.

2. Layer with chickpeas, avocado slices, mixed greens, and shredded carrots. Season with lemon juice, salt, and pepper to taste.

3. Roll the tortilla into a wrap and enjoy.

Gut-Healing Brown Rice and Veggie Bowl

Ingredients:

• 1 cup cooked brown rice

• 1 cup mixed sautéed vegetables (e.g., zucchini, bell peppers, mushrooms)

• 1/2 cup cooked and shredded chicken breast or tofu (optional)

• 1 tablespoon olive oil

• 1 tablespoon balsamic vinegar

• Fresh basil or parsley for garnish

• Salt and pepper to taste

Instructions:

1. In a bowl, combine cooked brown rice, sautéed vegetables, and shredded chicken or tofu (if using).

2. Drizzle with olive oil and balsamic vinegar. Season with salt and pepper.

3. Garnish with fresh basil or parsley before serving.

Gut-Healthy Lentil and Vegetable Stew

Ingredients:

- 1 cup dried green or brown lentils, rinsed

- 1 onion, diced

- 2 carrots, diced

- 2 celery stalks, diced

- 1 zucchini, chopped

- 4 cups vegetable broth

- 1 teaspoon ground turmeric

- 1 teaspoon ground cumin

- Salt and pepper to taste

- Fresh cilantro for garnish

Instructions:

1. In a large pot, sauté the onion, carrots, celery, and zucchini until they soften. Add the lentils, vegetable broth, ground turmeric, and ground cumin.

2. Bring to a boil, then reduce heat and simmer for about 25-30 minutes or until the lentils are tender. Season with salt and pepper.

3. Garnish with fresh cilantro before serving.

Gut-Healing Spinach and Strawberry Salad

Ingredients:

• 2 cups fresh spinach leaves

• 1 cup sliced strawberries

• 1/4 cup crumbled feta cheese (optional)

• 1/4 cup chopped walnuts

• Balsamic vinaigrette dressing: 2 tablespoons balsamic vinegar, 1 tablespoon olive oil, and 1 teaspoon honey (optional)

• Salt and pepper to taste

Instructions:

1. In a large bowl, combine fresh spinach, sliced strawberries, and crumbled feta cheese (if using). Sprinkle with chopped walnuts.

2. In a small bowl, whisk together balsamic vinegar, olive oil, and honey (if using).

3. Drizzle the dressing over the salad and season with salt and pepper.

Gut-Healthy Miso Soup

Ingredients:

• 4 cups water

• 2 tablespoons miso paste (white or red)

• 1 cup sliced mushrooms

• 1 cup chopped bok choy or spinach

• 1/2 cup cubed tofu

• 2 green onions, sliced

• 1 sheet nori (seaweed), torn into small pieces

• Soy sauce or tamari (optional, for extra flavor)

Instructions:

1. In a pot, bring water to a simmer.

2. In a small bowl, dilute the miso paste with a little warm water to form a smooth mixture.

3. Add the diluted miso paste, sliced mushrooms, bok choy or spinach, tofu, green onions, and torn nori to the simmering water.

4. Simmer for about 10-15 minutes or until vegetables are tender.

5. Adjust the flavor with soy sauce or tamari if desired.

Gut-Friendly Mediterranean Salad with Hummus

Ingredients:

• 2 cups mixed greens (e.g., romaine, arugula)

• 1/2 cup cherry tomatoes, halved

• 1/4 cup cucumber, diced

- 1/4 cup red onion, thinly sliced

- 1/4 cup Kalamata olives

- 2 tablespoons hummus for dressing

- Fresh lemon juice, olive oil, salt, and pepper for seasoning

Instructions:

1. In a bowl, combine mixed greens, cherry tomatoes, cucumber, red onion, and Kalamata olives.

2. Drizzle hummus over the salad and toss to coat.

3. Season with fresh lemon juice, olive oil, salt, and pepper.

Gut-Healing Quinoa and Black Bean Salad

Ingredients:

- 1 cup cooked quinoa

- 1 cup canned black beans, drained and rinsed

- 1 cup diced red bell pepper

- 1/2 cup corn kernels (fresh, frozen, or canned)

- 1/4 cup chopped cilantro

- 2 tablespoons lime juice

- 2 tablespoons olive oil

- 1 teaspoon ground cumin

- Salt and pepper to taste

Instructions:

1. In a large bowl, combine cooked quinoa, black beans, diced red bell pepper, corn kernels, and chopped cilantro.

2. In a small bowl, whisk together lime juice, olive oil, ground cumin, salt, and pepper.

3. Drizzle the dressing over the salad and toss to combine.

Gut-Healthy Tuna Salad Bowl

Ingredients:

- 1 can (5 oz) water-packed tuna, drained

- 2 cups mixed greens (e.g., arugula, spinach)

- 1/2 cucumber, sliced

- 1/2 cup cherry tomatoes, halved

- 1/4 cup red onion, thinly sliced

- Lemon-tahini dressing: 2 tablespoons tahini, 1 tablespoon lemon juice, and 1-2 tablespoons water to thin

- Salt and pepper to taste

Instructions:

1. In a bowl, flake the drained tuna.

2. Add mixed greens, cucumber, cherry tomatoes, and red onion.

3. Drizzle with lemon-tahini dressing and season with salt and pepper.

Gut-Healing Minestrone Soup

Ingredients:

- 1 cup cooked whole wheat or gluten-free pasta

- 4 cups vegetable broth

• 1 can (15 oz) kidney beans, drained and rinsed

• 1 cup diced zucchini

• 1 cup diced carrots

• 1 cup diced celery

• 1 cup chopped spinach

• 1 teaspoon dried basil

• Salt and pepper to taste

• Grated Parmesan cheese (optional, for garnish)

Instructions:

1. In a large pot, bring vegetable broth to a simmer. Add cooked pasta, kidney beans, diced zucchini, carrots, celery, and dried basil.

2. Simmer for about 15-20 minutes or until the vegetables are tender.

3. Stir in chopped spinach and cook for a few more minutes. Season with salt and pepper.

4. Garnish with grated Parmesan cheese if desired.

Ingredients:

• 1 cup cooked quinoa

• 1 cup roasted mixed vegetables (e.g., sweet potatoes, broccoli, bell peppers)

• 1/2 cup hummus

• 2 tablespoons lemon juice

• 2 tablespoons chopped fresh parsley

• Olive oil for drizzling

• Salt and pepper to taste

Instructions:

1. In a bowl, layer cooked quinoa and roasted mixed vegetables. Drizzle with olive oil.

2. In a small bowl, whisk together hummus, lemon juice, salt, and pepper.

3. Drizzle the hummus dressing over the bowl. Garnish with chopped fresh parsley.

Gut-Friendly Chicken and Vegetable Stir-Fry

Ingredients:

• 1 boneless, skinless chicken breast, sliced

• 2 cups mixed stir-fry vegetables (e.g., broccoli, snap peas, bell peppers)

• 2 cloves garlic, minced

• 2 tablespoons low-sodium soy sauce or tamari

• 1 tablespoon sesame oil

• 1/2 teaspoon grated fresh ginger

• Cooked brown rice for serving

Instructions:

1. In a wok or large pan, heat the sesame oil over medium-high heat.

2. Add sliced chicken and cook until no longer pink. Stir in minced garlic and grated ginger.

3. Add the mixed stir-fry vegetables and cook until they're tender-crisp. Drizzle with soy sauce or tamari and stir well.

4. Serve the stir-fry over cooked brown rice.

Gut-Healing Sweet Potato and Chickpea Curry

Ingredients:

• 1 large sweet potato, peeled and diced

• 1 can (15 oz) chickpeas, drained and rinsed

• 1 onion, chopped

• 2 cloves garlic, minced

• 1 can (14 oz) diced tomatoes

• 1 can (14 oz) coconut milk

• 2 tablespoons curry powder

• 1 tablespoon olive oil

• Salt and pepper to taste

• Fresh cilantro for garnish

Instructions:

1. In a large pot, heat the olive oil over medium heat.

2. Add chopped onion and garlic, sauté until they're translucent. Stir in the sweet potato, chickpeas, diced tomatoes, coconut milk, and curry powder.

3. Bring to a boil, then reduce the heat and simmer for about 20-25 minutes or until the sweet potatoes are tender.

4. Season with salt and pepper. Garnish with fresh cilantro before serving.

Gut-Healthy Sardine and Avocado Toast

Ingredients:

• 2 slices of whole-grain or sourdough bread

• 1 can (3.75 oz) sardines, drained

• 1 ripe avocado, mashed

• Sliced red onion

• Lemon juice, salt, and pepper for seasoning

Instructions:

1. Toast the bread until crisp. Spread the mashed avocado evenly on the toast.

2. Top with sardines and sliced red onion.

3. Season with lemon juice, salt, and pepper to taste.

Gut-Healing Cauliflower and Turmeric Soup

Ingredients:

• 1 head of cauliflower, chopped

• 1 onion, diced

• 2 cloves garlic, minced

• 1 can (14 oz) coconut milk

• 4 cups vegetable broth

• 1 teaspoon ground turmeric

- Olive oil for cooking

- Salt and pepper to taste

- Fresh parsley for garnish

Instructions:

1. In a large pot, sauté the diced onion and minced garlic in olive oil until they soften.

2. Add the chopped cauliflower, vegetable broth, and ground turmeric.

3. Bring to a boil, then reduce heat and simmer for about 15-20 minutes or until the cauliflower is tender.

4. Stir in the coconut milk. Use an immersion blender or regular blender to puree the soup until smooth.

5. Season with salt and pepper. Garnish with fresh parsley before serving.

Gut-Healthy Tofu and Broccoli Quinoa Bowl

Ingredients:

- 1 cup cooked quinoa

- 1 cup steamed broccoli florets

- 1/2 cup cubed tofu

- 2 tablespoons soy sauce or tamari

- 1 tablespoon sesame oil

- 1 teaspoon grated fresh ginger

- Sliced green onions for garnish

- Sesame seeds (optional)

Instructions:

1. In a bowl, combine cooked quinoa, steamed broccoli, and cubed tofu.

2. In a small bowl, whisk together soy sauce or tamari, sesame oil, and grated ginger. Drizzle the sauce over the bowl.

3. Garnish with sliced green onions and sesame seeds if desired.

Ingredients:

• 1 whole-grain or gluten-free tortilla

• 1/2 cup hummus

• 1/2 cup cucumber, sliced

• 1/2 cup cherry tomatoes, halved

• 1/4 cup Kalamata olives, pitted

• 1/4 cup feta cheese, crumbled (optional)

• Fresh mint leaves for garnish

Instructions:

1. Warm the tortilla in a dry skillet or microwave for a few seconds. Spread a layer of hummus on the tortilla.

2. Layer with cucumber slices, cherry tomatoes, Kalamata olives, and crumbled feta cheese (if using).

3. Garnish with fresh mint leaves. Roll the tortilla into a wrap and enjoy.

Gut-Healing Grilled Salmon with Quinoa and Asparagus

Ingredients:

• 2 salmon fillets

• 1 cup quinoa

• 1 bunch of asparagus, trimmed

• 2 tablespoons olive oil

• Lemon zest and juice

• Fresh dill, chopped

• Salt and pepper to taste

Instructions:

1. Preheat the grill to medium-high heat.

2. Brush the salmon and asparagus with olive oil, and season with salt and pepper.

3. Grill the salmon for about 4-5 minutes per side until cooked through, and grill the asparagus for about 3-4 minutes.

4. Cook quinoa according to package instructions.

5. In a bowl, combine cooked quinoa, lemon zest, lemon juice, and fresh dill.

6. Serve the grilled salmon and asparagus over the quinoa mixture.

Gut-Healthy Chickpea and Vegetable Stir-Fry

Ingredients:

• 1 can (15 oz) chickpeas, drained and rinsed

• 2 cups mixed stir-fry vegetables (e.g., broccoli, bell peppers, snap peas)

• 2 cloves garlic, minced

• 2 tablespoons low-sodium soy sauce or tamari

• 1 tablespoon sesame oil

• 1/2 teaspoon grated fresh ginger

• Cooked brown rice for serving

Instructions:

1. In a wok or large pan, heat the sesame oil over medium-high heat.

2. Add the mixed stir-fry vegetables and sauté until they're tender-crisp. Stir in minced garlic and grated ginger.

3. Add the chickpeas and cook for a few more minutes. Drizzle with soy sauce or tamari and stir well.

4. Serve the stir-fry over cooked brown rice.

Gut-Healing Spaghetti Squash with Pesto and Cherry Tomatoes

Ingredients:

• 1 spaghetti squash

• 1 cup cherry tomatoes, halved

• 2 tablespoons pesto sauce

• Fresh basil leaves for garnish

• Olive oil for drizzling

• Salt and pepper to taste

Instructions:

1. Preheat the oven to 375°F (190°C).

2. Cut the spaghetti squash in half lengthwise, remove the seeds, and place it cut-side down on a baking sheet.

3. Roast the squash for 30-40 minutes or until the flesh easily shreds with a fork.

4. Using a fork, shred the spaghetti squash into "noodles."

5. In a pan, heat the olive oil, add cherry tomatoes, and sauté until softened. Mix in the pesto sauce and season with salt and pepper.

6. Serve the pesto and tomato mixture over the spaghetti squash. Garnish with fresh basil leaves.

Gut-Friendly Black Bean and Vegetable Tacos

Ingredients:

• 1 can (15 oz) black beans, drained and rinsed

• 1 cup mixed sautéed vegetables (e.g., bell peppers, zucchini, onions)

- 1 teaspoon ground cumin

- 1 teaspoon chili powder

- 6 small whole-grain or corn tortillas

- Salsa, guacamole, and shredded lettuce for topping

Instructions:

1. In a pan, heat the sautéed vegetables, black beans, ground cumin, and chili powder until heated through.

2. Warm the tortillas in the oven or microwave. Fill the tortillas with the black bean and vegetable mixture.

3. Top with salsa, guacamole, and shredded lettuce.

Gut-Healthy Roasted Chicken and Vegetables

Ingredients:

- 4 bone-in, skin-on chicken thighs

- 1 pound baby potatoes

- 1 bunch of broccoli, cut into florets

- 1 lemon, sliced

- 4 cloves garlic, minced

- 2 tablespoons olive oil

- Fresh rosemary or thyme

- Salt and pepper to taste

Instructions:

1. Preheat the oven to 425°F (220°C).

2. In a large bowl, toss the chicken thighs, baby potatoes, broccoli, lemon slices, and minced garlic with olive oil, fresh rosemary or thyme, salt, and pepper.

3. Arrange the mixture on a baking sheet. Roast for 30-40 minutes or until the chicken is cooked through, and the vegetables are tender.

4. Serve the roasted chicken and vegetables hot.

Gut-Healing Lentil and Vegetable Curry

Ingredients:

- 1 cup dried green or brown lentils, rinsed

- 1 onion, chopped

- 2 cloves garlic, minced

- 1 can (14 oz) diced tomatoes

- 1 can (14 oz) coconut milk

- 2 tablespoons curry powder

- 2 cups mixed vegetables (e.g., carrots, bell peppers, peas)

- 2 tablespoons olive oil

- Salt and pepper to taste

- Fresh cilantro for garnish

Instructions:

1. In a large pot, sauté the chopped onion and minced garlic in olive oil until they soften.

2. Stir in the curry powder and cook for another minute. Add the lentils, diced tomatoes, coconut milk, and mixed vegetables.

3. Bring to a boil, then reduce the heat and simmer for about 20-25 minutes or until the lentils are tender.

4. Season with salt and pepper. Garnish with fresh cilantro before serving.

Gut-Healthy Baked Cod with Roasted Vegetables

Ingredients:

• 2 cod fillets

• 1 cup cherry tomatoes

• 1 cup asparagus spears

• 1 cup bell peppers, sliced

• 2 tablespoons olive oil

• Lemon zest and juice

• Fresh thyme or oregano

• Salt and pepper to taste

Instructions:

1. Preheat the oven to 375°F (190°C).

2. In a baking dish, place the cod fillets, cherry tomatoes, asparagus, and sliced bell peppers.

3. Drizzle with olive oil, lemon zest, lemon juice, fresh thyme or oregano, salt, and pepper.

4. Bake for about 15-20 minutes or until the cod is cooked through and the vegetables are tender. Serve hot.

Gut-Healing Stuffed Bell Peppers

Ingredients:

• 4 bell peppers, tops removed and seeds removed

• 1 cup cooked brown rice

• 1 cup lean ground turkey or plant-based alternative

• 1 can (14 oz) diced tomatoes

• 1 cup black beans, drained and rinsed

• 1 teaspoon ground cumin

• 1 teaspoon chili powder

• Salt and pepper to taste

• Grated cheddar or dairy-free cheese (optional)

Instructions:

1. Preheat the oven to 375°F (190°C).

2. In a skillet, cook the ground turkey (or plant-based alternative) until browned.

3. Add the diced tomatoes, cooked brown rice, black beans, ground cumin, and chili powder. Season with salt and pepper.

4. Stuff the bell peppers with the mixture and top with grated cheddar or dairy-free cheese if desired.

5. Place the stuffed bell peppers in a baking dish and bake for about 25-30 minutes or until the peppers are tender and the cheese is melted.

Gut-Healthy Veggie and Tofu Stir-Fry

Ingredients:

• 1 cup extra-firm tofu, cubed

• 2 cups mixed stir-fry vegetables (e.g., broccoli, snap peas, bell peppers)

• 2 cloves garlic, minced

• 2 tablespoons low-sodium soy sauce or tamari

• 1 tablespoon sesame oil

• 1/2 teaspoon grated fresh ginger

• Cooked quinoa or brown rice for serving

Instructions:

1. In a wok or large pan, heat the sesame oil over medium-high heat.

2. Add the cubed tofu and cook until lightly browned. Stir in minced garlic and grated ginger.

3. Add the mixed stir-fry vegetables and cook until they're tender-crisp. Drizzle with soy sauce or tamari and stir well.

4. Serve over cooked quinoa or brown rice.

Ingredients:

• 2-3 medium zucchinis, spiralized into noodles

• 1/2 cup pesto sauce

• Cherry tomatoes, halved

• Pine nuts (optional)

• Salt and pepper to taste

Instructions:

1. In a pan, lightly sauté the zucchini noodles until they're just tender.

2. Toss the zucchini noodles with pesto sauce and season with salt and pepper. Top with cherry tomatoes and pine nuts.

3. Serve warm or cold.

Gut-Healing Miso-Glazed Tofu with Brown Rice and Broccoli

Ingredients:

• 1 block extra-firm tofu, pressed and cubed

- 1 cup brown rice, cooked

- 2 cups broccoli florets

- 2 tablespoons white miso paste

- 1 tablespoon honey or maple syrup

- 1 tablespoon rice vinegar

- 1 tablespoon sesame oil

- 1 teaspoon grated fresh ginger

- 2 cloves garlic, minced

- Sesame seeds for garnish

- Soy sauce or tamari (optional)

Instructions:

1. Preheat your oven to 400°F (200°C).

2. In a bowl, whisk together white miso paste, honey (or maple syrup), rice vinegar, sesame oil, grated ginger, and minced garlic.

3. Toss the cubed tofu in the miso mixture and place it on a baking sheet. Roast the tofu for about 25-30 minutes or until it's golden and crispy.

4. Steam the broccoli until tender.

5. Serve the miso-glazed tofu over cooked brown rice, top with steamed broccoli, and garnish with sesame seeds. Add soy sauce or tamari if desired.

Gut-Healthy Quinoa and Chickpea Stuffed Bell Peppers

Ingredients:

• 4 bell peppers, tops removed and seeds removed

• 1 cup cooked quinoa

• 1 can (15 oz) chickpeas, drained and rinsed

• 1 cup diced tomatoes

• 1/2 cup diced red onion

• 1 teaspoon ground cumin

• 1/2 teaspoon smoked paprika

• Salt and pepper to taste

• Grated cheddar or dairy-free cheese (optional)

Instructions:

1. Preheat the oven to 375°F (190°C).

2. In a bowl, combine cooked quinoa, chickpeas, diced tomatoes, diced red onion, ground cumin, smoked paprika, salt, and pepper.

3. Stuff the bell peppers with the mixture and top with grated cheddar or dairy-free cheese if desired.

4. Place the stuffed bell peppers in a baking dish and bake for about 25-30 minutes or until the peppers are tender and the cheese is melted.

Gut-Healing Chickpea and Sweet Potato Stew

Ingredients:

• 1 can (15 oz) chickpeas, drained and rinsed

• 2 sweet potatoes, peeled and diced

- 1 onion, chopped

- 2 cloves garlic, minced

- 1 can (14 oz) diced tomatoes

- 4 cups vegetable broth

- 1 teaspoon ground cumin

- 1 teaspoon paprika

- Olive oil for cooking

- Salt and pepper to taste

- Fresh cilantro for garnish

Instructions:

1. In a large pot, sauté the chopped onion and minced garlic in olive oil until they soften.

2. Add the sweet potatoes, chickpeas, diced tomatoes, vegetable broth, ground cumin, and paprika.

3. Bring to a boil, then reduce the heat and simmer for about 20-25 minutes or until the sweet potatoes are tender.

4. Season with salt and pepper. Garnish with fresh cilantro before serving.

Gut-Healthy Baked Chicken Breast with Quinoa and Steamed Broccoli

Ingredients:

• 2 boneless, skinless chicken breasts

• 1 cup quinoa

• 2 cups broccoli florets

• 2 tablespoons olive oil

• Lemon juice

• Fresh thyme or rosemary

• Salt and pepper to taste

Instructions:

1. Preheat the oven to 375°F (190°C).

2. Season the chicken breasts with olive oil, lemon juice, fresh thyme or rosemary, salt, and pepper.

3. Bake for about 25-30 minutes or until the chicken is cooked through. While the chicken is baking, cook quinoa and steam broccoli.

4. Serve the baked chicken over quinoa and with steamed broccoli.

Gut-Healing Minestrone Soup with Whole Wheat Bread

Ingredients:

• 1 cup cooked whole wheat pasta

• 4 cups vegetable broth

• 1 can (15 oz) kidney beans, drained and rinsed

• 1 cup diced zucchini

• 1 cup diced carrots

• 1 cup diced celery

• 1 cup chopped spinach

• 1 teaspoon dried basil

• Salt and pepper to taste

• Whole wheat bread for dipping

Instructions:

1. In a large pot, bring vegetable broth to a simmer.

2. Add cooked whole wheat pasta, kidney beans, diced zucchini, carrots, celery, and dried basil. Simmer for about 15-20 minutes or until the vegetables are tender.

3. Stir in chopped spinach and cook for a few more minutes. Season with salt and pepper.

4. Serve with slices of whole wheat bread for dipping.

Gut-Healthy Turkey and Veggie Stir-Fry

Ingredients:

• 1 cup ground turkey

• 2 cups mixed stir-fry vegetables (e.g., broccoli, snap peas, bell peppers)

• 2 cloves garlic, minced

• 2 tablespoons low-sodium soy sauce or tamari

- 1 tablespoon sesame oil

- 1/2 teaspoon grated fresh ginger

- Cooked quinoa or brown rice for serving

Instructions:

1. In a wok or large pan, heat the sesame oil over medium-high heat.

2. Add the ground turkey and cook until browned. Stir in minced garlic and grated ginger.

3. Add the mixed stir-fry vegetables and cook until they're tender-crisp. Drizzle with soy sauce or tamari and stir well.

4. Serve over cooked quinoa or brown rice.

Gut-Friendly Sushi Bowls

Ingredients:

- 2 cups cooked sushi rice

- 8 oz sushi-grade salmon or tuna, cubed

- 1 cucumber, sliced

- 1 avocado, sliced

- 1/4 cup pickled ginger

- 2 tablespoons low-sodium soy sauce or tamari

- Wasabi and sesame seeds (optional)

Instructions:

1. Divide the cooked sushi rice into bowls.

2. Arrange the cubed salmon or tuna, sliced cucumber, sliced avocado, and pickled ginger on top. Drizzle with low-sodium soy sauce or tamari.

3. Add wasabi and sesame seeds for extra flavor if desired.

4. Serve the sushi bowls cold.

Gut-Healing Quinoa and Black Bean Stuffed Peppers

Ingredients:

- 4 bell peppers, tops removed and seeds removed

- 1 cup cooked quinoa

- 1 cup black beans, drained and rinsed

- 1 cup corn kernels (fresh, frozen, or canned)

- 1/2 cup diced tomatoes

- 1 teaspoon chili powder

- 1/2 teaspoon cumin

- Salt and pepper to taste

- Grated cheddar or dairy-free cheese (optional)

Instructions:

1. Preheat the oven to 375°F (190°C).

2. In a bowl, mix cooked quinoa, black beans, corn, diced tomatoes, chili powder, cumin, salt, and pepper.

3. Stuff the bell peppers with the quinoa mixture.

4. Place the stuffed peppers in a baking dish. Cover with aluminum foil and bake for about 30-35 minutes.

5. Remove the foil, top with grated cheddar or dairy-free cheese if desired, and bake for an additional 10 minutes or until the peppers are tender.

Gut-Healthy Lemon and Garlic Shrimp with Zucchini Noodles

Ingredients:

• 1 pound large shrimp, peeled and deveined

• 2-3 medium zucchinis, spiralized into noodles

• 2 tablespoons olive oil

• 4 cloves garlic, minced

• Zest and juice of 1 lemon

• Fresh parsley for garnish

• Salt and pepper to taste

Instructions:

1. In a large skillet, heat olive oil over medium-high heat.

2. Add shrimp and minced garlic, cook until shrimp turn pink. Add lemon zest, lemon juice, salt, and pepper.

3. Add the zucchini noodles and sauté for a few minutes until they're just tender.

4. Garnish with fresh parsley and serve.

Gut-Healing Eggplant and Chickpea Curry

Ingredients:

• 1 large eggplant, cubed

• 1 can (15 oz) chickpeas, drained and rinsed

• 1 onion, chopped

• 2 cloves garlic, minced

• 1 can (14 oz) diced tomatoes

• 1 can (14 oz) coconut milk

• 2 tablespoons curry powder

• 2 tablespoons olive oil

• Salt and pepper to taste

• Fresh cilantro for garnish

Instructions:

1. In a large pot, sauté the chopped onion and minced garlic in olive oil until they soften.

2. Stir in the cubed eggplant, chickpeas, diced tomatoes, coconut milk, curry powder, salt, and pepper.

3. Bring to a boil, then reduce the heat and simmer for about 20-25 minutes or until the eggplant is tender.

4. Garnish with fresh cilantro before serving.

Gut-Healthy Miso-Glazed Salmon with Brown Rice and Steamed Asparagus

Ingredients:

• 2 salmon fillets

• 1 cup cooked brown rice

• 1 bunch of asparagus, trimmed

- 2 tablespoons miso paste

- 1 tablespoon honey

- 1 tablespoon low-sodium soy sauce or tamari

- Olive oil for brushing

- Sesame seeds (optional)

- Salt and pepper to taste

Instructions:

1. Preheat the oven to 375°F (190°C).

2. In a small bowl, whisk together miso paste, honey, low-sodium soy sauce or tamari, and a splash of water to make the glaze.

3. Brush the salmon fillets with olive oil and season with salt and pepper.

4. Place salmon on a baking sheet, spread the miso glaze on top, and bake for about 15-20 minutes or until the salmon is cooked through. While the salmon is baking, steam asparagus until tender.

5. Serve the salmon with brown rice and steamed asparagus.

6. Garnish with sesame seeds if desired.

Gut-Friendly Butternut Squash and Spinach Salad with Quinoa

Ingredients:

• 2 cups cooked quinoa

• 2 cups cubed roasted butternut squash

• 2 cups fresh spinach leaves

• 1/4 cup dried cranberries

• 1/4 cup crumbled feta cheese (optional)

• Balsamic vinaigrette dressing: 2 tablespoons balsamic vinegar, 1 tablespoon olive oil, and 1 teaspoon honey (optional)

• Salt and pepper to taste

Instructions:

1. In a bowl, combine cooked quinoa, cubed roasted butternut squash, fresh spinach, dried cranberries, and crumbled feta cheese (if using).

2. In a small bowl, whisk together balsamic vinegar, olive oil, and honey (optional).

3. Drizzle the dressing over the salad and season with salt and pepper.

Gut-Healthy Greek Yogurt Parfait

Ingredients:

• 1 cup Greek yogurt (plain, unsweetened)

• 1/2 cup fresh berries (e.g., strawberries, blueberries)

• 1/4 cup granola

• 1 tablespoon honey (optional)

• Chopped nuts (e.g., almonds, walnuts) for garnish

Instructions:

1. In a glass or bowl, layer Greek yogurt, fresh berries, and granola.

2. Drizzle with honey if desired.

3. Garnish with chopped nuts for extra flavor and texture.

Gut-Healing Chia Seed Pudding

Ingredients:

• 3 tablespoons chia seeds

• 1 cup unsweetened almond milk (or any preferred milk)

• 1/2 teaspoon pure vanilla extract

• Fresh fruit (e.g., sliced bananas, berries) for topping

• Honey or maple syrup for sweetness (optional)

Instructions:

1. In a bowl, mix chia seeds, almond milk, and vanilla extract.

2. Cover and refrigerate for at least 4 hours or overnight until it thickens.

3. Serve with fresh fruit on top and drizzle with honey or maple syrup if you'd like.

Gut-Healthy Banana and Oat Cookies

Ingredients:

• 2 ripe bananas, mashed

• 1 cup rolled oats

- 1/4 cup unsweetened applesauce

- 1/4 cup chopped nuts (e.g., walnuts)

- 1/4 cup raisins or dried cranberries

- 1/2 teaspoon ground cinnamon

- 1/2 teaspoon pure vanilla extract

- Pinch of salt

Instructions:

1. Preheat the oven to 350°F (175°C).

2. In a bowl, combine mashed bananas, rolled oats, applesauce, chopped nuts, raisins or dried cranberries, ground cinnamon, vanilla extract, and a pinch of salt.

3. Drop spoonfuls of the mixture onto a baking sheet lined with parchment paper.

4. Bake for about 15-20 minutes or until the cookies are golden brown.

5. Let them cool before enjoying.

Gut-Healing Mixed Berry Smoothie

Ingredients:

• 1 cup mixed berries (e.g., strawberries, blueberries, raspberries)

• 1/2 cup Greek yogurt (plain, unsweetened)

• 1/2 cup unsweetened almond milk (or any preferred milk)

• 1 tablespoon honey (optional)

• Ice cubes

Instructions:

1. In a blender, combine mixed berries, Greek yogurt, almond milk, honey (if desired), and a few ice cubes.

2. Blend until smooth.

3. Pour the smoothie into a glass and enjoy.

Gut-Friendly Baked Apples with Cinnamon

Ingredients:

• 4 apples, cored and halved

- 2 tablespoons honey

- 1 teaspoon ground cinnamon

- Chopped nuts (e.g., almonds, pecans) for garnish

- Greek yogurt (optional)

Instructions:

1. Preheat the oven to 350°F (175°C).

2. In a bowl, mix honey and ground cinnamon. Brush the honey and cinnamon mixture over the apple halves.

3. Place the apples in a baking dish and bake for about 30-40 minutes or until they're soft.

4. Serve with a sprinkle of chopped nuts and a dollop of Greek yogurt if desired.

Gut-Healing Berry and Almond Butter Smoothie Bowl

Ingredients:

- 1 cup mixed berries (e.g., blueberries, raspberries, blackberries)

- 1/2 cup Greek yogurt (plain, unsweetened)

- 2 tablespoons almond butter

- 1/4 cup granola

- Chia seeds and fresh mint for garnish

Instructions:

1. In a blender, combine mixed berries, Greek yogurt, and almond butter. Blend until smooth.

2. Pour the smoothie into a bowl. Top with granola, chia seeds, and fresh mint.

3. Enjoy your creamy smoothie bowl!

Gut-Healthy Chocolate Avocado Mousse

Ingredients:

- 2 ripe avocados

- 1/4 cup unsweetened cocoa powder

- 1/4 cup honey or maple syrup

- 1/2 teaspoon pure vanilla extract

- A pinch of salt

- Fresh berries for garnish

Instructions:

1. In a blender or food processor, combine avocados, cocoa powder, honey or maple syrup, pure vanilla extract, and a pinch of salt.

2. Blend until smooth and creamy.

3. Divide the mousse into serving cups and chill in the refrigerator.

4. Serve with fresh berries on top.

Gut-Healing Coconut and Chia Seed Popsicles

Ingredients:

- 1 can (14 oz) coconut milk

- 3 tablespoons chia seeds

- 2 tablespoons honey or maple syrup

- 1/2 teaspoon pure vanilla extract

- Fresh fruit (e.g., kiwi slices, mango chunks)

Instructions:

1. In a bowl, mix coconut milk, chia seeds, honey or maple syrup, and pure vanilla extract.

2. Add fresh fruit to popsicle molds. Pour the coconut mixture into the molds.

3. Freeze for a few hours or until the popsicles are set.

4. Enjoy a refreshing and gut-friendly frozen treat.

Gut-Friendly Baked Pears with Cinnamon and Walnuts

Ingredients:

- 4 ripe pears, halved and cored

- 2 tablespoons honey

- 1 teaspoon ground cinnamon

- 1/4 cup chopped walnuts

• Greek yogurt (optional)

Instructions:

1. Preheat the oven to 375°F (190°C).

2. In a bowl, mix honey and ground cinnamon. Brush the honey and cinnamon mixture over the pear halves.

3. Place the pears in a baking dish and sprinkle with chopped walnuts. Bake for about 25-30 minutes or until the pears are tender.

4. Serve with a dollop of Greek yogurt if desired.

Gut-Healthy Blueberry and Oat Crisp

Ingredients:

• 2 cups fresh or frozen blueberries

• 1 cup old-fashioned oats

• 1/4 cup almond flour

• 1/4 cup chopped nuts (e.g., pecans)

• 2 tablespoons honey

- 2 tablespoons coconut oil

- 1/2 teaspoon ground cinnamon

- A pinch of salt

- Greek yogurt (optional)

Instructions:

- Preheat the oven to 350°F (175°C).

- In a bowl, combine blueberries and honey.

- In another bowl, mix oats, almond flour, chopped nuts, coconut oil, ground cinnamon, and a pinch of salt.

- Spread the blueberries in a baking dish and top with the oat mixture.

- Bake for about 30-35 minutes or until the crisp is golden and the blueberries are bubbling.

- Serve with a dollop of Greek yogurt if desired.

Gut-Healing Mango and Coconut Chia Popsicles

Ingredients:

- 1 cup ripe mango, diced

- 1 cup coconut milk

- 3 tablespoons chia seeds

- 2 tablespoons honey or maple syrup

- Popsicle molds

Instructions:

1. In a blender, blend the ripe mango until smooth.

2. In a bowl, mix the mango puree, coconut milk, chia seeds, and honey or maple syrup.

3. Pour the mixture into popsicle molds. Freeze for a few hours or until the popsicles are set.

4. Enjoy a tropical and gut-friendly frozen dessert.

Gut-Healthy Cinnamon and Almond Baked Apple Slices

Ingredients:

- 2 apples, cored and sliced

- 2 tablespoons almond butter

- 1/2 teaspoon ground cinnamon

- Chopped almonds for garnish

- Greek yogurt (optional)

Instructions:

1. Preheat the oven to 375°F (190°C).

2. In a bowl, mix almond butter and ground cinnamon.

3. Toss the apple slices in the almond butter and cinnamon mixture.

4. Place the apple slices on a baking sheet. Bake for about 15-20 minutes or until the apples are tender.

5. Serve with chopped almonds and a dollop of Greek yogurt if desired.

Gut-Healing Berry and Yogurt Popsicles

Ingredients:

• 1 cup mixed berries (e.g., strawberries, blueberries, raspberries)

• 1 cup Greek yogurt (plain, unsweetened)

• 2 tablespoons honey or maple syrup

• Popsicle molds

Instructions:

1. In a blender, blend the mixed berries, Greek yogurt, and honey or maple syrup until smooth.

2. Pour the mixture into popsicle molds. Freeze for a few hours or until the popsicles are set.

3. Enjoy these creamy and gut-friendly frozen treats.

Gut-Friendly Chocolate-Dipped Strawberries

Ingredients:

• Fresh strawberries

• Dark chocolate (70% cocoa or higher)

• Chopped nuts (e.g., almonds, pistachios)

• Shredded coconut (optional)

Instructions:

1. Wash and dry the strawberries.

2. Melt the dark chocolate in a microwave or on a stovetop with a double boiler.

3. Dip each strawberry into the melted chocolate, allowing excess chocolate to drip off.

4. Place the chocolate-dipped strawberries on a parchment paper-lined tray.

5. Sprinkle with chopped nuts or shredded coconut (if desired).

6. Allow the chocolate to set before serving.

Gut-Healthy Oatmeal and Banana Cookies

Ingredients:

• 2 ripe bananas, mashed

• 1 cup rolled oats

• 1/4 cup unsweetened applesauce

- 1/4 cup raisins or dried cranberries

- 1/2 teaspoon ground cinnamon

- 1/2 teaspoon pure vanilla extract

- A pinch of salt

Instructions:

1. Preheat the oven to 350°F (175°C).

2. In a bowl, combine mashed bananas, rolled oats, applesauce, raisins or dried cranberries, ground cinnamon, vanilla extract, and a pinch of salt.

3. Drop spoonfuls of the mixture onto a baking sheet lined with parchment paper.

4. Bake for about 15-20 minutes or until the cookies are golden brown.

5. Let them cool before enjoying these delicious and gut-friendly cookies.

Ingredients:

• 1 cup mixed berries (e.g., strawberries, blueberries, blackberries)

• 1 cup Greek yogurt (plain, unsweetened)

• 2 tablespoons honey or maple syrup

• Popsicle molds

Instructions:

1. In a blender, combine mixed berries, Greek yogurt, and honey or maple syrup until smooth.

2. Pour the mixture into popsicle molds. Freeze for a few hours or until the popsicles are set.

3. Enjoy these creamy and gut-friendly frozen popsicles.

Gut-Healthy Pineapple and Mint Sorbet

Ingredients:

• 2 cups fresh pineapple chunks

- Juice of 1 lime

- Fresh mint leaves

- 2-3 tablespoons honey or maple syrup (adjust to taste)

- A pinch of salt

Instructions:

1. In a blender, combine fresh pineapple chunks, lime juice, honey or maple syrup, and a pinch of salt. Blend until smooth.

2. Transfer to a container and freeze for about 4-6 hours.

3. Serve with fresh mint leaves for a refreshing and gut-friendly sorbet.

Gut-Friendly Baked Peaches with Cinnamon and Almonds

Ingredients:

- 4 ripe peaches, halved and pitted

- 2 tablespoons honey

- 1 teaspoon ground cinnamon

• 1/4 cup chopped almonds

• Greek yogurt (optional)

Instructions:

1. Preheat the oven to 375°F (190°C).

2. In a bowl, mix honey and ground cinnamon. Brush the honey and cinnamon mixture over the peach halves.

3. Place the peaches in a baking dish and sprinkle with chopped almonds.

4. Bake for about 20-25 minutes or until the peaches are tender.

5. Serve with a dollop of Greek yogurt if desired.

Gut-Healing Banana and Walnut Ice Cream

Ingredients:

• 3 ripe bananas, sliced and frozen

• 1/4 cup unsweetened almond milk (or any preferred milk)

• 1/4 cup chopped walnuts

• 1 teaspoon pure vanilla extract

• Honey or maple syrup for sweetness (optional)

Instructions:

1. In a blender, combine frozen banana slices, almond milk, chopped walnuts, pure vanilla extract, and honey or maple syrup (if desired). Blend until creamy.

2. Serve immediately for a delicious and gut-friendly ice cream.

Gut-Healthy Orange and Carrot Sorbet

Ingredients:

• 2 large carrots, peeled and chopped

• Juice and zest of 2 oranges

• 2-3 tablespoons honey or maple syrup (adjust to taste)

• Fresh mint leaves for garnish

Instructions:

1. In a blender, combine chopped carrots, orange juice, orange zest, and honey or maple syrup. Blend until smooth.

2. Transfer to a container and freeze for about 4-6 hours.

3. Serve with fresh mint leaves for a cool and gut-friendly sorbet.

CHAPTER THREE

In conclusion, embarking on a journey towards gut recovery is a profound investment in one's overall well-being. The intricate interplay between our gastrointestinal system and overall health cannot be overstated. Through this comprehensive guide, we have delved into the intricacies of gut health, exploring its anatomy, functions, and the pivotal role of the gut microbiome.

We've examined common digestive issues, their symptoms, and potential root causes. Understanding these factors empowers individuals to make informed choices about their lifestyle, diet, and overall wellness. The profound impact of diet on gut health has been underscored, with a focus on gut-friendly foods, fiber, probiotics, and prebiotics, as well as foods to limit or avoid.

Lifestyle factors, including stress management and exercise, play an equally significant role in maintaining a healthy gut. Consulting a healthcare professional for personalized guidance and advice is strongly encouraged, as they can offer tailored solutions and treatments. With practical steps and a structured gut recovery plan, individuals can take charge of their digestive health, fostering a flourishing gut environment. From reintroducing foods to tracking progress, this guide provides the tools necessary for a holistic approach to gut recovery.

Incorporating gut-friendly recipes for breakfast, lunch, dinner, and dessert adds a delightful dimension to this journey. These recipes are designed to nourish the gut while delighting the palate, proving that achieving gut health need not come at the expense of culinary enjoyment.

In essence, gut recovery is a journey towards equilibrium, where the delicate balance of our gastrointestinal system is nurtured and sustained. It's a journey towards vitality, comfort, and a profound sense of well-being. By embracing the principles outlined in this guide, individuals can embark on a path of holistic health that extends far beyond the digestive system, ultimately leading to a fuller, more vibrant life. Remember, a healthy gut is the cornerstone of overall wellness, and it's never too late to start on the path to recovery. Here's to a happy, healthy gut and a thriving you!